THE
SMOOTHIE
RECIPE BOOK
for Beginners

ESSENTIAL SMOOTHIES *to*
GET HEALTHY, LOSE WEIGHT,
and **FEEL GREAT**

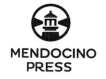

**MENDOCINO
PRESS**

Contents

PART TWO

Smoothie Recipes   53

Introduction

Health experts constantly remind us that we are sorely lacking fresh fruits and vegetables in our daily diets, and unfortunately for the majority of us, it's true. Perhaps this deficiency occurs because we're often busy, or maybe it's because heavily processed prepackaged foods are often the most convenient option available. Perhaps it's simply because we're not quite sure what to do with various kinds of produce.

Whatever our reasons for consuming fewer fresh fruits and vegetables than we should, there is ample evidence that increasing whole plant food intake is beneficial. People who focus on consuming an abundance of fresh produce each day are better able to ward off illnesses, have an easier time losing excess weight or maintaining a healthy body weight, and generally possess a healthy glow.

One of the easiest, most convenient ways to increase the amount of fresh plant foods you consume each day is to drink smoothies on a regular basis. With the help of this book, you'll discover not only how to make your own perfectly portable smoothies at home, but also how to speed up the process so you'll never have to miss breakfast or choke down another artery-clogging fast-food meal again.

Each of the wonderful smoothie recipes in this book has been created with great taste and optimum nutrition in mind, and each includes information about benefits imparted by specific ingredients. Whether you hope to lose weight, increase your energy level naturally, improve your looks, or eliminate toxins, smoothies can play an important part. Even the icy, refreshing dessert recipes come with an abundance of health benefits.

From selecting the right blender, shopping for ingredients, and incorporating superfoods, to undertaking a three- or seven-day smoothie cleanse complete with an easy-to-follow meal plan, you'll find that *The Smoothie Recipe Book for Beginners* has all the information you need to make smoothies an enjoyable addition to your healthy lifestyle.

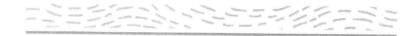

PART ONE

Smoothie Basics

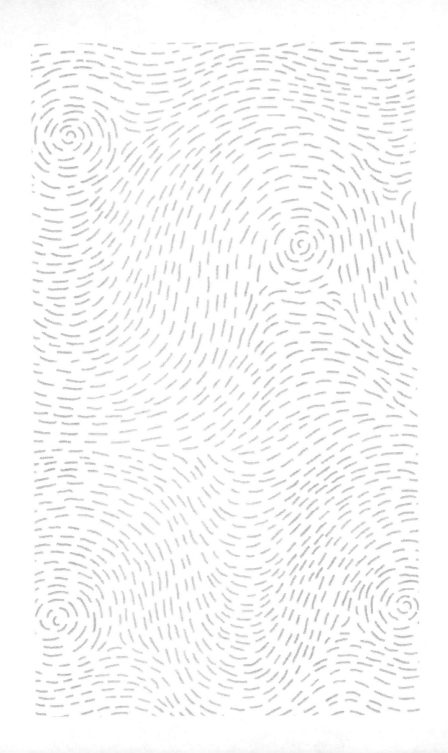

CHAPTER ONE

Why Drink Smoothies?

Most people want to eat more healthfully, but many have no idea where to begin. If you're trying to incorporate more fresh fruits and vegetables into your diet, you might find it difficult to do so, partly because chewing all of those plant products takes time, and partly because fresh foods can sometimes be hard to come by at venues other than supermarkets and farmers' markets. Plus, when those fresh options are available at restaurants and juice bars, they're often overpriced.

Smoothies are a quick, easy solution to all of these problems. The blender does the hard work of grinding up the fresh fruits and vegetables so that you can consume them in just a few minutes if you need to, and smoothies are wonderfully portable. You can shop for ingredients well in advance and store them. Finally, your budget won't suffer a bit when you make fresh smoothies at home; buying in-season produce and using the tips that follow will prevent you from overspending on premade options. As an added benefit, you'll know exactly what goes into each smoothie you make, ensuring that there are no unwanted additives like high-fructose corn syrup, artificial flavors, artificial colors, or other chemicals that do nothing to benefit your health.

SMOOTHIES VERSUS JUICES

When focusing on increasing your fruit and vegetable intake, you will undoubtedly encounter an abundance of data about the benefits of fresh juices and smoothies. While fresh juices are an excellent source of nutrition, there are several ways in which they differ from smoothies.

First, smoothies contain more fiber than juices do because smoothies consist of whole, raw fruits and vegetables rather than only the juice. This provides quite a few benefits, such as:

- Fiber keeps the digestive tract clear, allowing nutrients to be absorbed by the body and preventing complications such as constipation, diverticulitis, and the formation of hemorrhoids.
- Sugar is absorbed at a slow, even pace when adequate fiber is present in the foods we eat, preventing the spikes and subsequent crashes that happen when high-sugar, low-fiber foods are consumed.
- Fiber is bulky and takes some time to pass through the stomach, promoting feelings of fullness and preventing overeating.

Second, most smoothies keep well in the refrigerator, oxidizing much slower than juices do. While it's important to drink smoothies while they are fresh, they can be refrigerated in sealed containers for twenty-four to thirty-six hours; most juices need to be consumed immediately after they are made.

Third, smoothies are ideal for use as meal replacement shakes. While you cannot add an avocado, nuts, or seeds to a juicer and obtain the healthful fats that they contain, they are very easy to add to the blender, as are other robust ingredients such as raw cocoa nibs, medicinal herbs, and protein powders. You can also add tofu, yogurt, dairy milk, soy milk, nut milk, oat milk, or rice milk to your smoothies to increase nutrition; the options are endless.

Smoothies are nutritious, delicious, and fun to make. While the same may be said of juices, smoothies offer some benefits that juices do not, and since they're made in blenders, which are easier to clean than juicers, they offer greater convenience than fresh homemade juices do. Finally, since smoothies use whole fruits and vegetables, you don't need to use as much to fill up your glass, meaning you'll spend less on smoothies than you would on the same volume of fresh juices.

Making Fresh Juices to Add to Smoothies

If you already have a juicer, you can put it to good use by creating fresh juices to add to your smoothies. These juices are often superior to those found in supermarkets, as they contain only pure, natural ingredients. Consider making juices and freezing them in ice cube trays for later use. This will save you time while increasing the nutritional value of your smoothies.

HEALTH BENEFITS OF SMOOTHIES

Smoothies are incredibly versatile, and as you'll soon discover, it's very easy to incorporate many daily nutritional requirements into any recipe. You know that you should be getting plenty of vitamin C every day and that you ought to be taking in healthy omega-3 fatty acids. You may want to incorporate algae, seaweed, or some other unpalatable superfood into your diet, and you may wish to increase your intake of healthy fermented foods. With smoothies, you can do all of the above and more simply by adding the supplements you need most into the recipes that appeal to your taste. Fresh fruits have the ability to mask other flavors, making it simple to optimize nutrition while enjoying tastes that sometimes seem quite decadent.

Providing your body with the nutrition it needs leads to numerous health improvements, including:

- Better digestion
- Increased energy without the need for caffeine
- Reduced risk of chronic illnesses such as diabetes, hypertension, and heart disease
- Improved bone strength and decreased risk of osteoporosis
- Increased mental clarity

While no smoothie is a panacea, it's possible to incorporate ingredients that can aid in preventing some health problems and treating others. Before the advent of modern medicine, people often treated common maladies with food and herbs. And now, despite the availability of therapeutic drugs, many people continue to prefer natural treatments, either alone or in concert with medication. Some health benefits associated with smoothies and the ingredients they contain include:

- **Arthritis relief.** Consuming ginger in a smoothie can provide relief from pain and swelling associated with arthritis.
- **Blood pressure regulation.** Consuming whole plant foods in lieu of processed foods that contain high levels of salt can aid in reducing high blood pressure.
- **Reduced risk of stroke.** Decreasing blood pressure also decreases the risk of stroke. In addition, certain fruits such as apples and pears contain compounds that have been linked to a decreased stroke risk.
- **Prevent type 2 diabetes.** Due to the high level of magnesium they contain, leafy greens such as kale, collards, spinach, and even mild-tasting lettuce have been associated with a reduction in the risk of type 2 diabetes.
- **Eliminate headaches.** Many headaches are associated with stress, which can be exacerbated by an unhealthy diet. Consuming an abundance of fruits and vegetables each day can help cut down on headaches, including persistent migraines.

- **Reduce cold symptoms.** The common cold is caused by a virus and includes symptoms including a runny nose, cough, congestion, sore throat, and sneezing. The foods you consume while fighting a cold can help to reduce these symptoms and may also speed recovery. Smoothies are high in vitamin C, which is associated with these benefits.
- **Eliminate acne.** A diet high in B-complex vitamins and vitamin A is beneficial to skin health and can help to eliminate acne. Many fruits and vegetables contain high levels of these essential nutrients, and smoothies make it easy to ensure that you're getting enough to make a difference in the way your skin looks.
- **Ease seasonal allergy symptoms.** There are lots of natural remedies for seasonal allergies, many of which are easy to add to any smoothie recipe. Local honey, garlic, apple cider vinegar, turmeric powder, and poppy seeds are just a few supplements that can be incorporated into smoothies. As an added benefit, eating a diet high in vitamins and minerals strengthens the immune system, increasing resistance to allergies and other common health complaints.
- **Clear nasal congestion.** Congestion isn't just annoying—it can lead to painful pressure. Hot spices such as cayenne, horseradish, and wasabi can help reduce congestion, bringing rapid relief. They are very easy to incorporate into smoothies and are particularly appealing when added to green smoothie recipes that contain only vegetables.
- **Ease nausea.** There are many conditions that cause nausea, and while eliminating this symptom won't cure you, it can make you feel much more comfortable so you can rest while your body heals. Fresh or powdered ginger root is a well-known remedy for nausea and can be added to any smoothie recipe.

Beyond their ability to contribute to improved physical health, smoothies can also help boost self-confidence. When you focus on giving your body the best, little problems that can chip away at self-esteem often evaporate. Whether you feel insecure because you're overweight or because your skin has a tendency to break out, making smoothies part of your daily intake can help to eliminate these problems so you feel better about your appearance.

SMOOTHIES FOR WEIGHT LOSS

Unfortunately, an overabundance of convenience foods paired with time- and labor-saving technologies has contributed to an overwhelming problem with obesity. Whether you have just a few pounds to lose or you're severely overweight, you'll find that consuming smoothies on a regular basis makes it much easier to slim down.

Many diets simply call for a reduction in calories, while other plans focus on increased physical activity as the best way to lose weight. The truth is that both caloric intake and exercise play important roles in healthy weight loss—and so does nutrition. With smoothies, you maintain a balanced, healthy diet while enjoying the same level of convenience that may have led you to consume unhealthy fast foods that contributed to your weight gain. Like less healthful options, they are filling and very easy to enjoy while on the go.

Smoothies are simple to prepare ahead of time, package, and transport. When you've got a delicious, healthy meal close at hand while at work or traveling, the likelihood that you'll find yourself consuming unhealthy fast foods at your desk or behind the wheel decreases greatly. And here's a bonus: The more smoothies you drink, the less you will desire addictive fast foods and the more you will come to crave fresh, healthy plant foods.

All of the smoothie recipes in this book are suitable for inclusion in a weight loss plan, as they are high in fiber and relatively low in calories. Some, particularly those in the Dessert Smoothies chapter, are meant for occasional enjoyment, since they are much richer than others; however, they are still nutritionally superior to high-fat desserts containing unhealthy additives.

You can easily make any smoothie into a complete meal by adding some protein and a small amount of healthy fat to it. Incorporating a serving of tofu, yogurt or, dairy-free yogurt, milk or non-dairy milk, nuts, or nut butter is an excellent way to bulk up recipes that contain only fruits and vegetables.

It's just as easy to transform a rich smoothie into one with fewer calories and little or no fat. You can do this by cutting back on the amount of calorie-laden ingredients it contains; some simple ways to do this include replacing milk with green or herbal tea or using half a banana instead of a whole one—the average banana contains 110 calories, so using just half makes a difference. Nuts, nut butters, and avocados are worth including in your diet, but they should be enjoyed in moderation. Cut back if you need to lose weight.

Hunger causes many dieters to stray. Low-calorie smoothies, particularly green smoothies that incorporate leafy greens and other low-sugar vegetables with tasty fruits, satisfy hunger better than some high-calorie snacks do. By replacing unhealthy snacks such as cookies, donuts, and potato chips with smoothies, you can eliminate hundreds of calories from your diet while increasing feelings of satisfaction.

Cravings are another cause of diet derailment. Most often caused by deficiencies, cravings are rapidly eliminated when you give your body what it needs in terms of vitamins, minerals, and other nutrients. If you're trying to eliminate sugar addiction or a habit of constantly reaching for salty snacks, you'll need to focus on making good nutrition a priority. This is often difficult for the first few days, but stick with it, and you'll soon be craving healthful foods rather than those that contribute to obesity and the numerous health complications that go along with it.

SMOOTHIES FOR BEAUTY

Whether you're a woman with dry, brittle hair and nails or a man who is beginning to experience male pattern baldness—or simply someone with a desire for that naturally beautiful glow some people possess— drinking smoothies on a regular basis can provide your body with the nutrition it needs to look its very best.

Just like all other body tissues, hair, nails, and skin are composed mainly of protein, but they need additional nutrients to grow as well as to glow. When the body is deprived of essential nutrients, it focuses on maintaining the brain, the eyes, and other essential organs that are necessary for survival, leaving the hair and nails brittle and weak. Poor circulation related to inadequate nutritional intake leaves the skin looking pale, dry, and lifeless.

When you drink smoothies on a regular basis, you nourish every single cell of your body. While your organs will benefit, so will your hair, skin, and nails. Even if your intent isn't to improve your appearance, you'll find that this is likely to happen.

Leafy greens are among the many fruits and vegetables that contain B-complex vitamins, which are absolutely essential for vibrant-looking hair. Chili peppers and bananas are also excellent sources of these nutrients.

Vitamin C benefits your appearance by improving blood circulation, which in turn leads to a glowing complexion and increased blood flow to the tiny vessels that supply your hair follicles. With improved circulation comes faster hair growth. Citrus fruits, sweet and hot chili peppers, guava, broccoli, kiwi fruit, and dark leafy greens are some examples of smoothie ingredients that contain high levels of vitamin C.

Essential fatty acids including omega-3 and omega-6 are important for overall health and also have an impact on appearance. Without enough essential fatty acids in your diet, you'll suffer from dry and itchy skin, brittle nails, and hair that lacks shine and vitality. Flaxseed, pumpkin seeds, and walnuts are just a few examples of ingredients that contain the essential fatty acids required for good looks and great health.

Antioxidants contribute to appearance by protecting the body from free radicals that contribute to visual signs of aging. Dark red fruits and vegetables such as beets, blueberries, and pomegranates contain high levels of antioxidants, as do some other ingredients such as chia seeds.

SMOOTHIE FAQS

What exactly is a smoothie?

A smoothie is a drink, shake, or meal replacement that is made by processing whole fruits and vegetables in a blender, along with other ingredients such as milk, yogurt, tea, or juice. Smoothies can be sweet or savory, healthy or decadent; it all depends on what you add to the blender.

How thick should my smoothies be?

Smoothies are quite a bit thicker than plain juices are, but there is no set consistency to adhere to. Thickness is mostly a matter of personal preference—what is most important is that you enjoy the smoothies you make. They can be thinned for easier drinkability by adding water, tea, or other liquid, or they can be thickened by adding ice, which will slow the rate of consumption.

My smoothies are often too frothy. Is there a way to prevent or reduce foam?

Some high-pectin fruits such as apples and pears produce an abundance of froth when blended into smoothies. Try using a lower speed to reduce the amount of foam these fruits produce, or simply skim the foam off with a spoon or spatula before pouring the smoothie into your glass.

Sometimes my smoothie ends up curdling. Why is this happening? Is there a way to prevent it?

Certain smoothies have a tendency to curdle, particularly if they are made with dairy milk or yogurt and a high-acid fruit such as citrus or berries. The longer these combinations sit before consumption, the greater the likelihood that curdling will occur. Drinking your smoothie right away is one way to prevent unsightly curdling; using a non-dairy liquid is another.

Where can I buy superfoods? I haven't noticed them at the supermarket.

Superfoods like chia seeds, flaxseed, blue-green algae, chlorella, and others can be tough to find in supermarkets. If you have a health food store in your area, check to see if they have what you're looking for. If not, they may be able to order it for you. You can also buy superfoods from online retailers—but shop with a reputable dealer to ensure that you're getting the right product and that it's fresh and potent.

Can I add a sweetener to my smoothie?

If the smoothies you're making aren't sweet enough, you can certainly add more fruit to sweeten them. You can also add a natural sweetener such as maple or birch syrup, honey, agave syrup, brown rice syrup, or stevia extract. Avoid artificial sweeteners and refined sugars.

Should I ever substitute ingredients?

Substitution is definitely encouraged. Smoothies aren't like many other foods that call for precise ingredients; instead, they often work well with ingredients other than those a recipe calls for. Oranges, tangelos, and tangerines are wonderfully interchangeable, as are papayas, peaches, and mangos. If you have strawberries on hand but a recipe calls for raspberries or blueberries, there's no need to go back to the store; most berries are interchangeable as well.

Why do most smoothie recipes call for bananas?

Bananas give smoothies a creamy texture and plenty of body, and they're very easy to find in most places. If you don't have bananas or dislike their flavor, try making recipes without them. To reduce sugar in any recipe that calls for banana, simply use $\frac{1}{2}$ cup of yogurt, non-dairy yogurt, or well-drained tofu instead. However, you may need to use additional fruit or natural sweetener to improve palatability if you make this kind of substitution.

I don't do soy. Can I use something else in recipes that call for soy products?

It's very easy to use other products in place of soy. Yogurt can stand in for tofu, while hemp milk, almond milk, oat milk, rice milk, or dairy milk work well in place of soy milk.

I want to enjoy the benefits of wheatgrass in my smoothie. Can I add wheatgrass to the blender?

Wheatgrass does not do well in the blender, nor does it process well in a standard juicer. The best way to get the benefits of wheatgrass is to either use a wheatgrass supplement or use a wheatgrass juicer to make fresh wheatgrass juice to add to your smoothies.

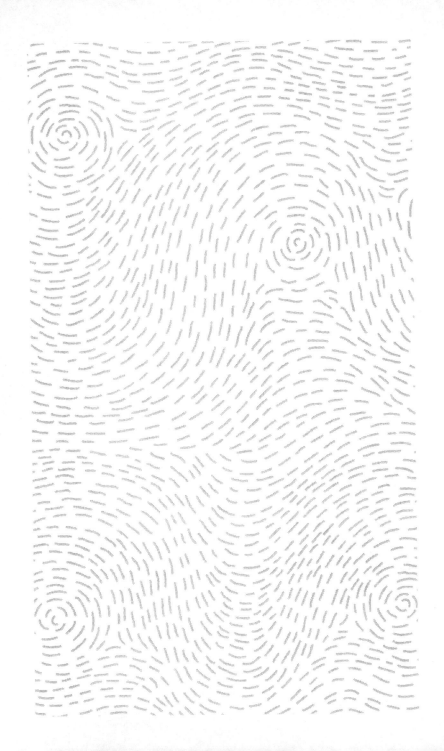

CHAPTER TWO

Getting Started with Smoothies

Smoothies are among the simplest foods to prepare using ordinary fruits and vegetables. You'll need to ensure that you have a few basic tools on hand before you start, and once you've assembled them, you won't need anything else unless you decide you'd like to upgrade. No matter which recipe you choose to try first, and no matter how often you plan to make smoothies, you'll need many of the same items, including a blender.

Once you have all the tools you need and you're ready to begin in earnest, simply use the advice in the shopping guide that follows to find the freshest ingredients available and perhaps save a little money while you're at it. After bringing fresh produce home from the market, refer to the preparation, storing, and freezing tips in this chapter to reduce waste, enhance the flavors and textures of your smoothies, and make your creations fast, fun, and as simple as possible.

KITCHEN TOOLS AND EQUIPMENT

If you normally prepare food at home, you probably have many of the tools you'll need to prepare fruits and vegetables for smoothies. If you're missing any of these tools, you can easily purchase them online or at a store that carries housewares.

Cutting Boards

There are many different types of cutting boards available; some are made of glass, others are made with tough plastic, and still others are made with various types of wood. Select a cutting board that is capable of withstanding heavy use and does not have a slippery surface—glass cutting boards are attractive, but they're probably the worst choice for prepping juicy foods that have a tendency to slip.

If possible, select a cutting board with a channel around its edge; this will catch excess drips and make cleanup much easier.

Finally, be sure that you only use the cutting board you choose for preparing fresh produce. Keep it away from fish, poultry, meat, and other items that could potentially spread bacteria. This is extremely important since all the ingredients you'll be adding to your smoothies will be raw.

Knives

You might think that very sharp knives are more dangerous than moderately sharp ones, but the exact opposite is true. Select sharp, heavy-duty knives that you can re-sharpen as needed. While these do often cost more than other options, they are capable of withstanding heavy use, cutting through tough rinds, and generally making the task of prepping fruits and vegetables faster and easier.

There are a few types of knives you'll want to assemble, since different food items call for different preparation techniques. These include:

- A serrated slicing knife for preparing fruits with soft skins.
- A paring knife for cutting blemishes and tough peels away from produce, and for slicing fruits into small pieces to save wear and tear on your blender.

- A chef's knife or French knife for cutting through large fruits and vegetables. Choose one with a heavy handle.
- A utility knife, which is ideal for working with medium-size fruits and vegetables.

If you don't have a knife sharpener, it's a good idea to get one. Be sure to watch a few online tutorials about sharpening knives or, better yet, have an experienced chef teach you how to do this simple task properly. Good knives are a worthwhile investment and can sometimes last for decades, but incorrect sharpening can ruin them.

Colander or Strainer

Washing is an essential part of preparing fresh produce for smoothies, and it's almost impossible to do a good job without a colander or strainer. Select a large-capacity model that's capable of accommodating a significant amount of food.

Salad Spinner

A salad spinner is a device meant for washing leafy greens and other lightweight produce such as blackberries, raspberries, blueberries, and grapes. It speeds up the preparation process and gets food squeaky clean.

Measuring Cups and Spoons

While any kind of measuring cups will work in a pinch, the best for smoothie preparation are large liquid measuring cups. These look a bit like small pitchers and are available in various models. Plastic measuring cups cost less, but those made of metal or glass last longer.

Any kind of measuring spoons will work. Most are made of plastic, but metal ones are also available.

Kitchen Shears

Kitchen shears are not an absolute necessity, but they make tasks like snipping fresh herbs, cutting through grape stems, and chopping small amounts of leafy greens faster and easier. Regular scissors will work in a pinch, but they won't last through more than a few washes.

Corers, Slicers, and Other Timesaving Food Prep Tools

Visit a home or kitchen store, and you'll find an amazing array of tools designed to significantly reduce produce preparation time. Melon ballers, vegetable peelers, spatulas, and special slicers are some options to look for.

Baking Sheets

Baking sheets are great for freezing fresh fruits for later addition to smoothies. While you can choose the simplest option available, be sure to select a size that will easily fit in your freezer.

Ice Cube Trays

One of the easiest ways to store liquid ingredients and pre-blended smoothies for later use is to freeze them. Using ice cube trays allows you to easily measure and monitor portions, and small cubes are much easier to handle than large lumps of frozen liquid.

HOW TO CHOOSE A BLENDER

If you've already got a countertop blender, you'll probably be able to use it to make smoothies. If not, you'll need to obtain a blender that is capable of crushing ice and reliably processing fruits and vegetables.

If possible, select a powerful blender designed for making smoothies. These generally cost more but are usually quieter, tend to last longer, and normally deliver superior results. These blenders have a multitude of settings including puree, whip, chop, grind, crush, and blend and are designed to withstand regular heavy use. They often come with excellent warranties that cover not just the motor but also the blades and other parts.

It's okay to purchase an inexpensive blender if you're not sure you'll be sticking with your smoothie habit or if your budget doesn't allow for a high-end blender. You can find countertop blenders for as little as $20, and you can certainly use them to create smoothies that are both healthful and delicious.

No matter what your budget, be sure to conduct plenty of research before settling on a blender. There are many online resources with feedback from people who have used the same blenders you are considering, and this kind of information can be just as useful as the product specifications provided by manufacturers and retailers.

There are several important things to consider when choosing a blender:

- Ensure that the blender's pitcher is glass or very strong plastic. Steer clear of cheap blenders with plastic pitchers.
- Choose a blender with a sharp, durable blade and a strong motor.
- Select a model with enough capacity to handle more than one smoothie at once. Preparing large quantities of smoothies ahead of time is a very good way to develop a good smoothie-drinking habit and stick with it.
- Look for preprogrammed speed options and be certain that the blender has the ability to crush ice. In addition, make sure it's equipped with a pulse function.

If you'd like a high-end blender but can't afford a brand-new one right away, don't overlook online auction sites like eBay. If you decide to buy a secondhand blender, be sure that the description and photos seem accurate, and make sure that you purchase from a seller with a good reputation. It's also possible to buy reconditioned blenders from retailers, including online stores, and you can sometimes purchase display models from brick-and-mortar stores at discounted prices. Even though you may be itching to get started making smoothies, it pays to use a careful approach when selecting your blender.

SHOPPING GUIDE

Eating the healthiest foods possible doesn't have to be difficult or expensive. When shopping for smoothie ingredients, follow these simple tips to save time, money, and effort.

Know Your Produce

Learn about the fruits and vegetables you plan to buy before you go shopping. In most cases, you'll want to look for produce that is brightly colored, fairly firm, and free of blemishes, soft spots, bruises, shriveling, or mold. Ripe fruit often has a lightly sweet smell, while spoiled produce often has a distinctly unpleasant odor. Use the following tips to make shopping for certain items easier.

BERRIES

Berries of all kinds should look plump and ripe, without excessive green spots. Be sure to flip berry containers over and inspect them; those that are going bad often have leaking juices, and sometimes mold is visible on berries that have been crushed.

CITRUS

Lemons, limes, oranges, and other citrus fruits should have bright, smooth skin, and they should be free of soft spots, brown spots, or wrinkles. The ripest, tastiest citrus fruits usually feel heavy for their size; very light fruits are often under-ripe or have begun to dry out.

GRAPES

Grapes are usually very easy to shop for; be sure to look for bunches with no obvious spoilage, and try to purchase organic grapes if possible, since conventional growers liberally dose them with pesticides and fungicides.

PEACHES

Peaches often look beautiful even when they don't taste good. To determine if peaches are ripe, hold them near your nose and breathe in. You should catch a whiff of fresh peach fragrance. If you don't want to rely on your sense of smell, look at the yellow areas on the peach; they should have vibrant color and no green spots. In addition, peaches should feel slightly heavy for their size, and they should give a little when you feel them. A peach that feels firm is not ripe, and one that feels very soft may be ripe and sweet but will need to be used immediately.

PINEAPPLE

Ripe pineapples smell delicious and are heavy for their size. Avoid those with soft spots or mold. If you can't find a ripe pineapple, choose an attractive green one. It will ripen nicely within a week.

Buy in Bulk

Whether you buy fresh or frozen produce to add to your smoothies, purchasing in bulk can save you money. As a bonus, stocking your freezer full of smoothie ingredients helps to keep its temperature even, saving you a little money on your monthly energy bill.

Buying in bulk saves time and money in another way, too. When you purchase plenty of ingredients to keep on hand, you'll ultimately spend less time shopping, and you'll make fewer trips to the store overall.

Select Seasonal Ingredients

Purchase ingredients when they are in season, particularly if you have access to a farmers' market that offers local produce. Either get exactly the quantity you need for a few smoothie recipes to avoid waste, or stock up and freeze ingredients for later use. Freezing your own smoothie ingredients does take a little time and effort, but it's a good way to make the most of the fresh foods that local growers have to offer.

Stock Up When Items Are on Sale

If a certain ingredient is on sale, stock up if you can. All smoothie ingredients can be frozen for future use, and you can even pre-make smoothies and freeze them for later.

Plan for Shopping Trips in Advance

Make a shopping list before you head to the market. This way, you won't forget to purchase ingredients for the recipes you want to make. Keep in mind that some items last longer than others; berries stay fresh for just a day or two in the refrigerator, while robust fruits like apples and oranges retain their freshness for well over a week in most cases. Keep an eye out for bargains, but don't buy more than you can reasonably use or process at once. It's extremely disheartening to pay for fresh produce only to end up losing it to spoilage.

FRESH VERSUS FROZEN

Many who are new to making smoothies wonder whether fresh fruit is superior to frozen fruit. If you grow your own fruit and can pop it into the blender immediately after harvesting it or if you forage for wild berries and can use them right away, this might be the case. It also might be true if you have easy access to freshly picked fruit from local farmers.

In many cases, produce found at supermarkets and other stores has been shipped for thousands of miles and placed in long-term cold storage before being offered for sale. While these fruits and vegetables offer an abundance of nutrition, they are sometimes inferior to frozen fruits in terms of flavor and nutritional content. Fruit that has been frozen and packaged prior to sale is usually picked at the peak of ripeness and processed almost immediately afterward.

As to whether fresh smoothie ingredients are better than frozen ones, it's largely a matter of personal preference. While fresh fruits often impart sweet, delicate flavor to smoothies, frozen fruit adds texture while offering equal or better nutrition, depending on the fruit. Plus, pre-frozen fruits have already been peeled and cut, meaning you have less work to do when you use frozen fruits in your smoothies. You can use fresh and frozen fruits interchangeably in all of the recipes in this book, as well as in smoothie recipes you find elsewhere.

PREPARATION TECHNIQUES

Not all fruits were created equal. Knowing how to properly prepare your produce is an essential step to making delicious smoothies and getting the most out of your fruits

- **Berries**—When you bring fresh berries home from the market, pick through them immediately and remove any damaged ones. To store in the refrigerator, place a paper towel in the bottom of a container and store the berries inside. Be sure the container is not airtight; berries need to breathe in order to remain fresh. Do not wash your berries until just before using or freezing them. When cleaning berries, remove any stems and be sure to eliminate all visible soil. Unless you have very large strawberries that you plan to freeze before adding to smoothies, there's no need to cut berries before adding them to the blender.

- **Cherries**—Unless you are using frozen cherries without pits, you will need to remove the pits from cherries before adding them to your blender. You can use a cherry pitting tool to do this, or you can cut the cherries in half and remove the pits. Do not add cherry stems to the blender; they should be discarded.

- **Citrus Fruits**—Citrus fruits should be peeled before you add them to the blender, and seeds should be removed. Removing the white pithy layer that lies just below citrus skin will prevent bitterness, but it also eliminates some of the fruit's nutrients, so consider leaving the pith intact to improve nutrition. Unless you plan to freeze citrus before adding it to recipes, there's no need to cut it before storing.

- **Grapes**—Grapes should be removed from their stems and washed thoroughly before being added to smoothies. There's no need to cut grapes; whether fresh or frozen, they can be added to the blender whole.

- **Mangos**—Mangos have a large, flat pit inside, and they are very slippery if peeled before slicing. Cut large slices from your mangos, then lay the slices flat and slide a paring knife between the fruit and skin. You can add large chunks of mango to your smoothies; if you plan to freeze this fruit, cut it in one-inch cubes for easy processing.

- **Peaches**—Peaches can be stored on the countertop until ripe, after which they can be placed in the refrigerator for up to a week. Wash them just before cutting; most peaches can be cut in half with ease, though some have sticky pits and will need to be cut into small slices. If you plan to freeze peaches, cut them into one-inch chunks to ensure easy processing later.

- **Pineapples**—If you purchase a pineapple that isn't quite ripe, store it on a trivet or cooling rack on the countertop so that air can circulate around it for complete ripening and less risk of spoilage. Ripening can take anywhere from two days to a week, so be sure to check your pineapple frequently. You'll know that it's ripe when its fragrance intensifies; it may also get heavier as it ripens.

To prepare fresh pineapple for addition to smoothies, cut the spiny top off then slice the pineapple into quarters. Cut the woody core away from each quarter, and then slice it into one-inch wedges. Cut the fruit away from the skin before adding it to the blender. Store excess pineapple in a sealed container inside the refrigerator for up to a week or cut the fruit into one-inch chunks and freeze for later use.

Ripen fruits naturally—*If you'd like to hasten fruit's natural ripening process, it is easy to do so. Simply place the fruit in a paper bag at room temperature, out of direct sunlight. Fold the top of the bag to keep it closed. To speed the process even more, put an apple or a banana into the bag with the other fruits. The natural ethylene the fruits produce will be trapped inside the bag and will cause them to ripen more rapidly than fruits stored in the refrigerator or on the countertop. After the fruit ripens, use it right away or store it in the refrigerator to prevent spoilage.*

STORING AND FREEZING TIPS

Making large batches of smoothies and storing them for later use saves time and reduces the amount of cleanup effort you'll need to expend.

Fresh smoothies can be stored in sealed containers inside the refrigerator for up to thirty-six hours. Separation happens frequently and is normal; simply stir the smoothie before pouring it into your glass and drinking it.

You can also store smoothies and smoothie ingredients in the freezer for later use, which saves time and prevents the discoloration due to oxidation that can sometimes happen in the refrigerator. Here are some handy techniques to try at home:

- **Freeze fresh fruits.** Cut fruits into one-inch pieces and spread on a cookie sheet covered with parchment paper. Leave in the freezer for twelve to twenty-four hours, then store in plastic freezer bags marked with the name of the fruit and the date it was frozen. Add fruit to smoothie recipes as needed.

- **Put frozen ingredients together for premade recipes.** Measure all of your solid smoothie ingredients and freeze on cookie sheets covered with parchment paper. Freeze liquid ingredients in ice cube trays. Once all ingredients are frozen, place them in freezer bags marked with the name of the smoothie recipe and the date it was assembled. When you're ready to enjoy a smoothie, simply add the contents of the bag to the blender with a little bit of water or other liquid and enjoy.

- **Freeze smoothies in ice cube trays.** Prepare smoothie recipes as directed, then pour them into ice cube trays, filling each compartment about three-quarters of the way. Cubes should freeze within twelve to twenty-four hours. Store cubes in plastic freezer bags marked with the name of the smoothie and the date it was frozen. Practice portion control by determining how many cubes a serving of smoothie makes; various ice cube trays hold different amounts, so this will vary from one tray to the next. To reconstitute, either pour cubes into a travel mug and allow them to melt as you sip during your morning commute, or make a frosty smoothie by reprocessing the cubes in the blender.

CHAPTER THREE

Five Steps to the Perfect Smoothie

While smoothies aren't foolproof, they're actually quite easy to make, particularly when you follow the five simple steps in this chapter. Whether you're experimenting with combinations of your own or using a recipe, you'll find that these steps are the keys to obtaining reliably consistent results.

To make the process as simple as possible, each of the recipes in the chapters that follow has been created for ease of use. All you need to do is to add the ingredients in the same order as they appear in the recipe.

This chapter explains each step of this tried-and-true method in detail; follow the steps, and the smoothies you make will rival those offered by top establishments. With just a little practice and some experience, you'll soon be able to whip up perfect smoothies without giving the procedures involved a second thought.

STEP ONE: PICK FRUITS AND VEGETABLES

It's true that you can add any fruit or vegetable to a smoothie, but it's also true that quality matters, not just in terms of flavor but also in terms of nutrition. When making smoothies, remember that the more frozen items you add, the less likely you'll need to add ice. Also, the juicier the ingredients, the less liquid you may need, but you may want to add more ice to give your smoothie the desired texture. Here are a few tips to help you choose your smoothie ingredients:

- You can use either fresh or frozen fruits and vegetables in your smoothies—it's mostly a matter of personal preference. If you live in a place where fresh fruits are abundant year-round, it may make more sense to purchase these. If you live in a remote area where fresh options are few and far between, frozen ingredients may be the most sensible choice.
- Fresh produce in season is always an excellent addition to a smoothie recipe, particularly if those fruits and vegetables were grown locally. Fresh produce that must be shipped long distances is often covered with a layer of protective wax that can be hard to remove, and it's often less flavorful than fresh, local choices.
- When selecting ingredients to add to your smoothies, try to choose as many organic fruits and vegetables as you can. Organic food is grown without pesticides and herbicides that harm the planet and increase the body's toxic load. At the very least, be sure to choose organic versions of these so-called "dirty dozen" for smoothies and cooking: apples, peaches, grapes, celery, cucumbers, spinach, sweet peppers, hot peppers, nectarines, cherry tomatoes, potatoes, and strawberries. (See www.ewg.org/foodnews for the Environmental Working Group's most current list.)
- Always choose the fruits and vegetables that look, feel, or smell the best. Get your senses involved in the selection process; even if you're a little unsure about what to look for in a specific fruit or vegetable, your instincts will steer you in the right direction.
- Almost everyone enjoys creating new smoothie combinations without following recipes to the letter. You can easily make your own tasty concoctions by looking at flavors others have combined in the past. Some places to look for inspiration include the supermarket's juice aisle, yogurt section, and even the candy department.

Consume a Rainbow of Fruits and Vegetables Daily

Ensure that you are providing your body with the best natural nutrition possible by consuming fruits and vegetables in every color of the rainbow each day. Different-colored plants contain high concentrations of certain essential nutrients:

- **Red**—Bright red fruits and vegetables are high in lycopene, which is noted for its ability to reduce arterial inflammation, scavenge free radicals, and even inhibit the formation of cancer cells.
- **Orange and yellow**—Carrots, sweet potatoes, citrus fruits, and other foods with orange or yellow coloration contain high levels of beta carotene, which helps to improve eye function and prevent common eye diseases while enhancing skin health and improving immune function.
- **Green**—Green plants contain high levels of chlorophyll, which aids in purifying the body and building healthy new blood cells. They're also high in essential carotenoids, including zeaxanthin and lutein, along with folate, copper, potassium, vitamin B-6, and magnesium.
- **Blue and purple**—Not only are blue and purple fruits and vegetables a beautiful addition to your diet, but also they're rich in phytochemicals, antioxidants, and flavonoids. These powerful foods also contain anthocyanins, which have the ability to minimize DNA damage and slow the progress of nonmalignant cancer cells.
- **White**—Onions, garlic, leeks, and scallions are examples of white foods that contain an antimicrobial compound called allicin, which destroys viruses, bacteria, and fungi. Allicin is also highly regarded for its anti-inflammatory action and has been linked to reduced cholesterol levels and improved heart and vascular health.

***Try fresh coconut**—Raw, fresh coconut is an amazing food that contains an abundance of nutrition. Its outer shell makes it intimidating to deal with, but once you get a coconut open, your efforts will be well rewarded. Begin by placing the coconut in a 350°F oven for twenty minutes. Afterward, set it aside until it is cool enough to be handled, and then place the tip of a clean flat-head screwdriver into one of the coconut's three indentations. Tap the screwdriver gently with a hammer to puncture the shell. Repeat the process with another indentation. After you've made a small hole in the coconut's flesh, turn it upside down over a bowl to allow the water inside to drain. Then place it on a flat, sturdy surface, hitting it with the hammer until it breaks in two. Hit each half of the shell with the hammer until the flesh pops loose and use your hands to break each half into smaller pieces. Use a paring knife to separate the coconut flesh from the brown inner rind, then slice or grate it for easy use.*

STEP TWO: CHOOSE A LIQUID

Every smoothie needs a liquid base, as liquid promotes even blending and prevents ingredients from getting stuck. Most recipes call for between 1/2 and 1 cup of liquid, but you can use more or less if you like, and you can freeze your favorite liquids to use in place of ice cubes in the smoothies you make. Some of the best liquids to try include the following:

- **Water**—Be sure to use clean, filtered water both for drinking and for making smoothies. There are usually chemicals in tap water, and bottled water often isn't much better.
- **Dairy milk**—If you include dairy products in your diet, you'll find that milk makes a good start for a wide variety of smoothies. It doesn't normally work well in recipes that call for highly acidic ingredients, however, since the acid can cause the milk to curdle.

- **Nondairy milk**—There are a variety of excellent nut milks available in supermarkets, and soy milk, oat milk, and rice milk are other options to try. These milks are typically low in cholesterol and high in protein; watch out for added sugar, and look for those that don't contain genetically modified (GMO) ingredients.
- **Tea**—Tea makes an excellent substitute for water in many smoothie recipes. You can use fruit-infused herbal teas for extra fruit flavor without increasing calories, or you can give your smoothie a caffeine boost and additional antioxidants by choosing black, green, or white tea. If you love coffee, you can use it in smoothies, too—just be sure to choose complementary flavors such as vanilla, chocolate, or cinnamon.
- **Juices**—Juices with no added sugar make great smoothie bases, particularly if you make them with your own juicer. Some juices that aren't easy or practical to make at home can be found at grocery and health food stores—these include acai and pomegranate juices. Customize flavors by blending your favorite juices with tea, or reduce calories by using half juice and half water in recipes that call for juice.
- **Greek yogurt**—Greek yogurt has been strained through a filter to remove most of the whey, so a single serving contains fifteen grams of protein, which is nearly twice the amount found in a serving of traditional yogurt. Choose a brand with no additives, and be sure to select one with active cultures, which are good bacteria that promote healthy digestion while strengthening your immune system.

STEP THREE: ADD HEALTHFUL EXTRAS

There are a number of healthful extras that can be added to smoothies to give them flavor or thickness while increasing nutritional value. Here are some of the best additions; let your imagination run wild and try other extras as you see fit.

- **Fermented extras**—Fermented foods aren't just delicious, they're also rich with enzymes that help to keep the beneficial bacteria living within the gastrointestinal system in balance. Dairy and nondairy yogurt make excellent additions to smoothies, as do kefir and kombucha.
- **Nuts and nut butters**—Make smoothies more filling and better tasting by adding your favorite nuts or nut butters to recipes. Both options contain fiber, protein, and healthful fat and can transform a snack into a wonderfully delicious meal replacement.
- **Seeds**—Seeds, including flaxseed, chia seeds, and others, provide a protein boost while increasing your recipe's omega-3 content. Grind or soak seeds before adding to smoothies to ensure that your body is able to access all the nutrients they contain.
- **Chlorophyll boosts**—Powdered wheatgrass and barley grass contain chlorophyll, which helps to balance blood pH levels, plus a plethora of vitamins, minerals, amino acids, enzymes, and antioxidants. Green algae powders including chlorella and spirulina are excellent sources of protein with an abundance of vitamins.
- **Healthful supplements**—Protein powder adds nutritional value and texture to smoothies, and vitamin powders, fiber powders, oats, bran, and other additives provide numerous benefits. There are many brands available in different flavors; choose one without artificial sweeteners, colors, or flavorings.
- **Protein powder**—You can add a scoop of protein powder to any smoothie recipe to transform it into a light meal or make a meal replacement shake even more filling. When shopping for protein powder, find a brand that suits your personal dietary needs; some are designed for those who want to gain or lose weight, while others are designed to provide basic nutrition.

Superfoods

Adding superfoods to your diet is a simple yet powerful step you can take to achieve optimal health. There are dozens of easy-to-find superfoods that you can add to your diet to maintain your weight, combat disease, reduce your risk of heart disease and cancer, lower your cholesterol, and even help enhance your mood. Everyday superfoods that are great for smoothies include blueberries, spinach, oranges, and oats. Some top superfoods that are less known include:

- **Acai berry**—Acai berries are grown in South America and are just as popular there as blueberries are in North America. They contain an abundance of antioxidants, fatty acids, and phytosterols that combat high cholesterol; in addition, consumption is linked to improved metabolism and better digestion.
- **Aloe vera**—Aloe vera is a succulent plant that can be used whole, as food-grade gel, or as juice. It boosts immunity, improves digestion, and can aid in alleviating chronic inflammation. It is also an excellent addition to cleansing and detoxifying smoothies, as it has a mild laxative property.
- **Bee pollen**—Bee pollen was used by ancient healers from Egypt to China, who documented its ability to rejuvenate the body. It contains high levels of protein, vitamins, and minerals, as well as vital trace elements and more than five thousand enzymes.

- **Blue-green algae**—Blue-green algae, also known as aphanizom-enon flos-aquae (AFA), is a complete superfood that contains every nutrient the human body requires. Some of the benefits it provides include improved brain function, increased energy, and mood stability.
- **Camu camu berry**—Camu camu berry has the highest known vitamin C content of any food source, along with numerous antioxidants that help to boost the immune system. It has been linked to improved eyesight and better brain function; in addition, it has antiviral properties that make it the perfect dietary supplement for use during cold and flu season. It's typically found in powder form and can be purchased at most health food stores.
- **Chia seeds**—Chia seeds may be tiny, but they are powerful. They contain protein, omega-3 fatty acids, and high levels of antioxidants.
- **Chlorella**—Chlorella is a single-celled algae and an excellent source of chlorophyll. Known for its detoxifying abilities, it's excellent for cleansing recipes. It can also help to improve digestion and boost the immune system.
- **Goji berries**—Goji berries have been used in Asian cuisine for more than five thousand years. Said to promote longevity and improve mood, these tiny red berries are usually dried for easy shipping. They contain high levels of vitamins, minerals, and antioxidants.
- **Hemp seeds**—Hemp seeds are very high in protein; in fact, hemp protein has all twenty amino acids and is highly digestible. Hemp seeds contain high levels of vitamin E, along with essential fatty acids and other micronutrients.
- **Kelp seaweed**—Kelp is an excellent source of iodine, which is essential for thyroid balance. In addition, it is a good source of vitamins and minerals. Usually added to smoothies in powdered form, it has a slightly salty taste that many find quite pleasing.

- **Maca root**—Maca root is a tuber sourced from the high Andes. Used for both food and medicine for more than two thousand years, it increases energy and improves physical endurance.
- **Marine phytoplankton**—Marine phytoplankton is a type of algae that grows in the ocean. It's an excellent alternative to fish oil due to its ability to supply long-chain omega-3 essential fatty acids and is an excellent source of vitamins and minerals. It's also known to act as an anti-inflammatory and is linked to improved circulatory health.
- **Spirulina**—Spirulina is a type of freshwater blue-green algae. This single-celled aquatic plant contains all eight essential amino acids, is high in protein, and is brimming with antioxidants, vitamins, and minerals. It's well known for its ability to promote healthy skin and hair.

Try algae—If you've been consuming the standard American diet for years, then your taste buds have become accustomed to intense flavors—salty, sweet, sour, and savory alike. Many people who are new to the concept of consuming superfoods, particularly algae, find themselves feeling a faint sense of disgust as they wonder what these beneficial foods will taste like. While some forms of algae have a strong flavor, chlorella, blue-green algae, and spirulina taste a bit like spinach—and they are very easy to disguise in smoothies, soups, and other foods that contain strong flavors. The more healthful, naturally-flavored foods you consume and the less often you eat foods containing artificial flavors and flavor enhancers like MSG, the less these plant flavors are likely to disturb you; you may even come to enjoy them. Start with a very small amount and work your way up to the recommended serving size if you like.

STEP FOUR: SPICE IT UP

Just as herbs and spices add zest to recipes for everyday foods, they add interesting flavor to smoothies. You can blend nearly any spice into a smoothie for a more appealing taste; herbs, natural sweeteners, and other special additions also provide extra flavor. Try:

- Spices
- Natural sweeteners
- Extracts and essential oils
- Herbs
- Flavor intensifiers
- Special "dessert" ingredients, such as ice cream or whipped topping

The Easy Way to Wash Fresh Herbs

Fresh herbs make excellent additions to green smoothies, but they are often grown in sandy soil that leaves residue behind. The easiest way to remove all of the sand from herbs such as parsley and cilantro is to soak the herbs in a large bowl filled with water, then swish them vigorously to dislodge particles of soil. Dump the soiled water from the bowl and repeat the process at least one more time, then pat the herbs dry with paper towels before removing their leaves and adding them to the blender.

Dislike Stevia? Try These Natural Sweeteners

Some forms of stevia leave a slight aftertaste. While most people either don't notice it or don't mind it, some individuals dislike it and prefer not to use stevia in any form. If you want to sweeten a smoothie or some other type of food, consider using any of the following sweeteners instead of refined sugar or an artificial sweetener.

- **Maple Syrup**—Pure maple syrup offers numerous health benefits, boosting the immune system, promoting heart health, and more. Choose organic maple syrup to reduce your risk of exposure to harmful toxins.
- **Raw Honey**—Raw honey contains high levels of antioxidants, helps promote healthy digestion, and provides many other health benefits. It is lower on the glycemic index than many other forms of sugar are, and it tastes marvelous in smoothies, on cereal or toast, and even in plain Greek yogurt. Be sure to choose honey from a local source rather than mass-produced honey from the supermarket, which is sometimes adulterated with cheap imitation sweeteners.
- **Date Sugar**—Though it's called "sugar," this form of sweetener isn't highly processed; instead, it is an extract sourced from nutritious dried dates. With essential minerals including calcium, zinc, iron, and selenium, it is linked to improved cognitive function, enhanced immunity, and improved blood pressure.

Avoid artificial sweeteners—Artificial sweeteners seem to be everywhere. Though they can be a helpful tool for those who must avoid sugar because of blood sugar concerns, they are not ideal for weight loss. These zero-calorie sweeteners increase your taste for carbohydrates and sweets. The chemicals they contain have been linked to numerous adverse side effects, and recent studies show that they may be linked to an increased risk of cancer. Instead of artificial sweeteners, try pure stevia extract. It is an excellent calorie-free alternative to artificial sweeteners, and thanks to an increase in popularity, this natural sweetener is easy to find in most supermarkets.

STEP FIVE: BLEND

Careful blending techniques yield superior smoothies. Instead of just tossing all the ingredients for a recipe into the blender, follow these five simple steps to ensure your smoothies are perfect every time.

1. Start by choosing the right blender for the job. Almost any blender will work, with the exception of hand-held immersion blenders, which are not able to crush ice or take on other heavy tasks. Bullet-style blenders intended for smoothies often work well, but they're not suitable for blending large batches.

2. Add liquid to the blender before you add any other ingredients. In recipes that call for a variable amount of liquid, begin with the smaller amount and add more liquid if needed. This will prevent you from creating a smoothie that's thinner than you'd like.

3. Add bananas and other soft fruits and vegetables to the liquid in the blender's reservoir. Alternately blend and pulse to ensure all ingredients are well incorporated and to ensure that no large chunks are sticking to the blades. Once the mixture is smooth, you're ready to add greens, ice, or any frozen ingredients the recipe calls for.

4. Add ice, frozen fruit, and other tough ingredients in small batches of about a handful at a time. This will prevent sticking and ensure that all ingredients are smoothly incorporated. Don't be alarmed if your smoothies don't turn out perfectly at first, particularly if you're working with a new blender. Once you have familiarized yourself with the blender, you'll find it's much easier to get desirable results quickly.

5. Finally, be sure to clean up right away. Follow the instructions that came with your blender, ensuring that you remove all debris from the blades, cleanse the pitcher thoroughly, and wipe the base well to remove spills that could cause damage to electronic components.

CHAPTER FOUR

Smoothie Cleanse

The standard American diet is heavily reliant on foods that are laden with sugar, gluten, artificial colors and flavors, and stimulants. Eliminating them can be done cold turkey, but it's easier on your body and your psyche to undergo the process of cleansing gradually.

During a smoothie cleanse, you make a commitment to consume only plant-based smoothies for a certain period of time. The goal is to help you end unhealthy habits and enhance the quality of your daily diet by increasing your intake of vegetables and fruits.

Whether you want to jump-start a healthy weight loss plan, reduce your risk of suffering from life-threatening illnesses, increase your lifespan, or simply look and feel better than you may have in quite some time, a smoothie cleanse can help you to achieve your goals.

By drinking one smoothie at a time, day by day, you will nourish your body at a cellular level while eliminating built-up toxins. Many people enjoy cleansing so much that they do it on a regular basis, usually monthly or quarterly. While it's possible to undergo extended cleansing periods, it's best to start slowly with a short cleanse lasting no more than three days.

WHAT'S A SMOOTHIE CLEANSE?

A smoothie cleanse is a period of time during which you eat and drink only smoothies, water, and herbal teas. A cleanse may last for just one day or much longer; some who are experienced with cleansing choose to take on cleanses lasting thirty days or more.

During a smoothie cleanse, it's important to recognize that your body will undergo some changes as toxins are released from deep within cellular structures. You may experience mild skin breakouts, headaches, and fatigue, particularly during the first few days of your first cleanse. The more often you cleanse, the less pronounced these side effects will become, particularly if you stick to a healthy eating plan and keep drinking smoothies between cleanses.

BENEFITS OF A CLEANSE

There are many reasons to undertake a smoothie cleanse. The main benefits include rapid, healthy weight loss; increased energy; and the ability to think more clearly. When you spend a few days consuming nothing but smoothies, herbal teas, and water, your system is flooded with phytonutrients, vitamins, and minerals in abundance. This helps your body stay strong and increases your ability to ward off illness.

If you're addicted to sugar and processed foods, as so many people are, a smoothie cleanse is an excellent way to eliminate harmful cravings and replace them with a desire for fresh, natural foods.

SHOULD I CLEANSE?

While a smoothie cleanse can help nearly anyone regain health and improve overall well-being, there are some people who should not cleanse. If any of the following apply to you, include smoothies in your daily diet rather than cleansing. You'll still enjoy the benefits without subjecting your body to potentially harmful stress.

- Pregnant or nursing women
- People who are underweight
- Those with a history of eating disorders including anorexia and bulimia

- People under eighteen years of age
- Insulin-dependent diabetics
- People with liver or kidney disease
- Anyone with an irreversible wasting disease such as advanced-stage AIDS or metastatic cancer
- Those with cardiovascular complications or vascular disease
- Anyone suffering from a severe manic-depressive condition requiring medication
- People who suffer seizures

There are many other medical conditions for which this type of cleansing is contraindicated. If you're on any type of prescription medication or if you have any doubts as to whether you are healthy enough to cleanse, be sure to talk with your doctor beforehand.

THREE-DAY SMOOTHIE CLEANSE

During a three-day smoothie cleanse, your body will rid itself of toxins just as it would on a traditional three-day water fast, but the process comes with side effects that are less pronounced and much easier to handle.

The following meal plan has been created using a variety of smoothie recipes found in the second part of this book, especially chapter six, "Smoothies for Health." Feel free to make substitutions as you see fit, but be sure to drink at least two green smoothies during each day of the cleanse, and use at least two different types of greens throughout the cleanse. It's easy to make any smoothie recipe into a green one—simply add a one- to two-cup serving of leafy green vegetables such as spinach, kale, or chard to the blender just before adding ice and any supplements you want to include.

Three-Day Smoothie Cleanse Meal Plan

Breakfast
Banana Energy Shake
Mid-Morning Snack
Green Berry Detox Blast
Lunch
Filling Avocado Freeze
Mid-Afternoon Snack
Purple Grape–Papaya Protection
Dinner
Carrot Cleanse

DAY TWO

Breakfast
Heart-Healthy Fruit and Oat Shake
Mid-Morning Snack
Melon-Mint Refresher
Lunch
Berry-Almond Body Builder
Mid-Afternoon Snack
Green Grape Greatness
Dinner
Happy Heart

DAY THREE

Breakfast
Wellness Wake-Up
Mid-Morning Snack
Ginger Detox Delight

Lunch
Tropical Muscle Machine
Mid-Afternoon Snack
Watermelon Wellness
Dinner
Chocolate-Cherry Champion

SEVEN-DAY SMOOTHIE CLEANSE

Over the course of a seven day smoothie cleanse, your body will undergo some dramatic changes, inside and out. During the first three days, toxins will be eliminated. By the fifth day, the process of healing the immune system and rebuilding damaged cellular structures will be well underway. By the seventh day, you'll be sleeping better than ever, and your thought process will be sharper, too.

While it's possible to undergo a seven-day cleanse without first working your way through a shorter three-day cleanse, many people find that it's much easier to accustom the body to the process of cleansing beforehand.

As with the three-day cleanse, feel free to make substitutions in the following meal plan, ensuring that you drink at least two green smoothies daily.

Seven-Day Smoothie Cleanse Meal Plan

DAY ONE

Breakfast
Honey-Banana Health Fix
Mid-Morning Snack
Spicy Tomato-Cucumber Cleanse

Lunch
Greek Protein Punch
Mid-Afternoon Snack
Mindful Melon
Dinner
Blueberry-Avocado Body Bliss

DAY TWO

Breakfast
Apple-Cinnamon Power Breakfast
Mid-Morning Snack
Mellow Mango
Lunch
Purple Protein Pick-Me-Up
Mid-Afternoon Snack
Green Love Machine
Dinner
Coconut Craving

DAY THREE

Breakfast
Nuts over Oatmeal Energy Shake
Mid-Morning Snack
Mango Enlightenment
Lunch
Green Banana Detox
Mid-Afternoon Snack
Melon Cleanse
Dinner
Chocolate-Cherry Champion

DAY FOUR

Breakfast
Oat-Berry Breakfast Breeze
Mid-Morning Snack
Protective Peaches and Greens
Lunch
Detox Dream
Mid-Afternoon Snack
Spicy Tomato-Cucumber Cleanse
Dinner
Gorgeous Green Machine

DAY FIVE

Breakfast
Hearty Banana-Flax Power Shake
Mid-Morning Snack
Spicy Tomato-Cucumber Cleanse
Lunch
Ravishing Raspberry Ripple
Mid-Afternoon Snack
Watermelon Wellness
Dinner
Banana-Avocado Tummy Tamer

DAY SIX

Breakfast
Pomegranate Protection
Mid-Morning Snack
Spicy Tomato-Cucumber Cleanse

Lunch
Peachy Banana Protein Power

Mid-Afternoon Snack
Watermelon Wellness

Dinner
Tofu Temptation

DAY SEVEN

Breakfast
Kiwi-Banana Belly Blaster

Mid-Morning Snack
Mango Miracle

Lunch
Berry-Vanilla Vitality

Mid-Afternoon Snack
Cucumber-Celery Power Cleanse

Dinner
Slender Sensation

BEFORE, DURING, AND AFTER A CLEANSE: TEN ESSENTIAL TIPS

It takes time for our bodies to become damaged; likewise, it takes time to build better health. The cleansing process isn't the easiest, but these tips can help make it less challenging.

1. **Prepare your system for cleansing.** Slowly weaning yourself off foods like meat, fish, and heavy carbohydrates, as well as sugar and substances like alcohol, coffee, and cigarettes, makes cleansing less shocking to your system. Give yourself a week or two to cut back while including smoothies in your everyday diet.

2. **Shop for essentials in advance.** Buy smoothie ingredients and other essentials before beginning your cleanse. Supermarkets are filled with tempting aromas and visual cues, and avoiding them will help to reduce the likelihood that you'll break your cleanse earlier than planned.

3. **Take time off.** Try to take some time off from work, at least for the first few days of your cleanse. Side effects, particularly on the first and second day, are likely to be fairly unpleasant and can include excess gas as well as a need to evacuate the bowels more often and more urgently than normal. If you can't take time away from work and other daily activities, be sure to gradually eliminate toxic substances from your diet while increasing your smoothie intake. Giving your body a few weeks to adjust can greatly reduce the most unpleasant and embarrassing side effects associated with cleansing.

4. **Drink plenty of water.** Most of us don't drink nearly enough water. Get into the habit of drinking at least eight 8-ounce glasses of water each day before your cleanse begins, and continue drinking plenty of water during and after cleansing. Water helps to facilitate the cleansing process as it carries toxins out of the body. Replacing other beverages with clean, filtered water is one of the best things you can do for your health.

5. **Get more sleep.** Sleep is vital to good health, as while you're asleep, important rejuvenation processes are in progress. Focus on getting at least seven to eight hours of sleep each night, and try to get even more than that during the cleansing process.

6. **Consume organic foods.** Conventionally grown foods contain toxic residues that can build up in your body over time, while organic foods are raised without chemical fertilizers, herbicides, or pesticides that could be detrimental to your health. Eating organic foods reduces your exposure to chemical toxins; without their interference, your body is able to function properly.

7. **Switch to natural products.** Gradually replace household cleaning products and personal hygiene products with natural products that don't contain noxious chemicals. Not only are these products better for the planet, but they're also better for your and your family's health.

8. **Learn to meditate.** Meditation isn't necessarily a religious practice, although there are many faith traditions that utilize it for spiritual reasons. Meditating enables you to become more attuned to the way your body is feeling and helps you focus your mind and relax. Even if you meditate for just ten to fifteen minutes per day, you'll enjoy less mental fatigue, lower blood pressure, and an improved ability to recognize and respond to your own physical and emotional needs.

9. **Exercise.** Many of us spend hours in sedentary postures, either by choice or because our jobs demand it. Even a little daily exercise can counteract all of the sitting while improving digestion, aiding in our ability to sleep well, and promoting overall wellness. If you're not currently exercising, start by walking for a few minutes daily and gradually increase the length and duration of your walks. Make gentle exercise such as yoga, swimming, or walking part of each day you cleanse. Keep your newly established habit after cleansing, and you'll notice improved physical, mental, and emotional well-being.

10. **Treat yourself.** Treating yourself doesn't necessarily mean consuming lots of heavy foods and less-than-healthy beverages. During your cleanse, treat yourself to the opportunity to do things you may not normally have time for. Spend time on your favorite hobbies, watch movies you've always wanted to see, and read books that inspire and enlighten you. Treat yourself to long baths, luxurious lotions, and extended catnaps. Not only will this help to ease any discomfort you experience during your cleanse, but it will also help you look forward to cleansing as a way to slow down and enjoy life a little more.

Enhance success by planning cleanse activities—*If you've ever spent time at a retreat, you know that although the activities that take place are often relaxing, they are well-planned. Planning your daily activities hour by hour may not be something you normally do, but structuring your days so that activities flow from one to the next can help you stay on track, keeping you focused and enhancing your success.*

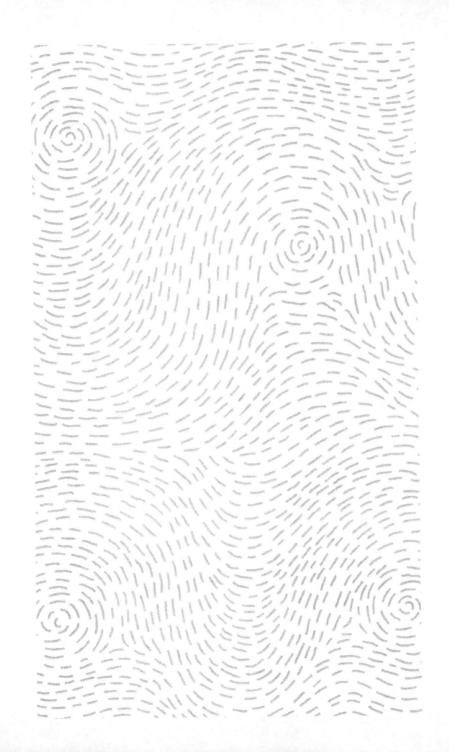

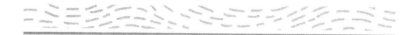

Smoothie Recipes

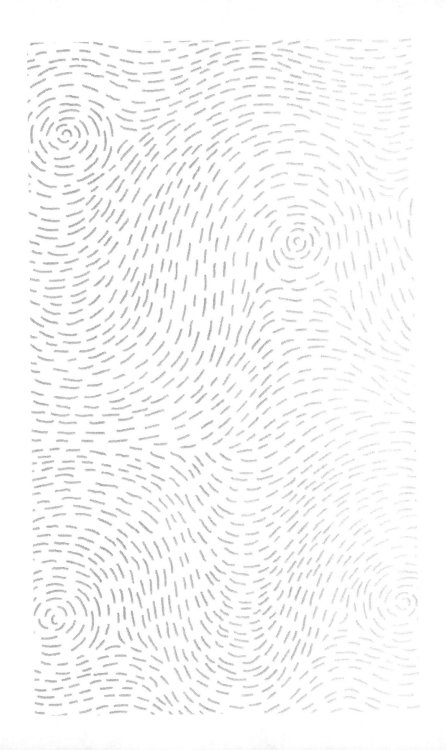

CHAPTER FIVE

Breakfast Smoothies

Despite the fact that breakfast is a very important meal—perhaps the most important of the day—many of us choose to eat a few quick sugary calories, opt for a fast-food meal from a drive-through, or worst of all, skip it altogether.

Eating breakfast does more than just prevent you from getting too hungry and bottoming out later in the day. It provides you with a mental advantage by preventing brain fog caused by fatigue and depleted glycogen stores. In addition, it makes you less vulnerable to succumbing to cravings for foods you're better off without.

Whether you're cleansing your body or simply drinking smoothies as a fast and easy way to improve your overall health, you'll find that the recipes in this chapter contain enough calories, fiber, and protein to get even the busiest day off to a good start. In contrast to quick fillers like sugary coffee drinks, pastries, and other typical breakfast foods, these healthful smoothies are designed to provide you with lasting energy and better nutrition while offering delicious flavors.

The fiber in each of these recipes helps to keep you feeling full for a few hours, and the protein nourishes your body's cells and promotes alertness. Whether you prepare the smoothies in advance or whip them up as you're beginning your morning, you'll soon find that it's difficult to go even one day without them. Many of the recipes in this chapter make large quantities, so you can share breakfast with someone special or save a portion or two for a later meal or snack.

***Eat between 350 and 500 calories at breakfast**—Breakfast revs metabolism, so even if you are trying to lose weight, it's important that you consume an entire meal's worth of calories each morning. Studies have repeatedly shown that people who eat a hearty breakfast feel less hungry during the rest of the day than those who eat little or no breakfast. Be sure that your breakfast—whether it's a smoothie or something else—contains protein, complex carbohydrates, and a small amount of healthy fat such as that found in almond milk, avocados, nuts, or seeds.*

Banana Energy Shake

▶ 62 CALORIES PER CUP

Bananas are sweet yet mild, and they give smoothies a creamy consistency that makes them a pleasure to drink. In addition, they contain high levels of vitamins, minerals, and antioxidants, and they offer an almost instant energy boost. Though fairly low in calories, this delightful smoothie is very high in vitamin C, thanks to the pineapple it contains. Unsweetened almond milk adds protein, ensuring that you remain satisfied for hours. You can add a superfood such as bee pollen to this smoothie for even more nutritional value.

1 CUP UNSWEETENED ALMOND MILK
1 BANANA, PEELED AND CUT INTO 1-INCH CHUNKS
2 CUPS FRESH PINEAPPLE CHUNKS
6 ICE CUBES

1. Pour the almond milk into the blender. Add the banana and blend until smooth.

2. Add the pineapple and process until well blended.

3. Add the ice cubes and blend until the desired consistency has been achieved.

4. Pour into a glass and enjoy.

Wellness Wake-Up

YIELDS 3 CUPS

▶ 87 CALORIES PER CUP

This delicious breakfast smoothie contains wheat germ and a banana for instant energy and an abundance of fiber. The sweet, juicy mango is an excellent source of vitamins C, A, and B-6, plus it contains beta carotene and trace minerals to promote healthy brain function.

Add a superfood supplement if you like, such as spirulina, goji berries, or protein-rich hemp seed. For an extra-icy treat, freeze the banana and mango before making your smoothie.

½ CUP UNSWEETENED ALMOND MILK
1 BANANA, PEELED AND CUT INTO 1-INCH CHUNKS
1 CUP FRESH MANGO CHUNKS
1 TABLESPOON WHEAT GERM
4 ICE CUBES

1. Pour the almond milk into the blender.

2. Toss the banana and mango together with the wheat germ and add them to the almond milk, then process until smooth and creamy.

3. Add the ice cubes, then blend and pulse until well incorporated.

4. Pour into a glass and enjoy.

Honey-Banana Health Fix

YIELDS 3 CUPS

▶ 110 CALORIES PER CUP

Honey is more than just a chemical-free natural sweetener; it's brimming with antioxidants and flavonoids that may help to reduce the risk of chronic diseases, including heart disease. Ancient Olympians ate dried figs and honey to improve athleticism, so there's no doubt that you can count on these high-energy ingredients to make your morning go smoothly.

If you prefer a brighter flavor, use freshly squeezed orange juice in place of the almond milk, but you may need to eat a few nuts to boost your protein intake for the morning.

1 CUP UNSWEETENED ALMOND MILK
1 BANANA, PEELED AND CUT INTO 1-INCH CHUNKS
¼ CUP DRIED FIG PIECES
1 TABLESPOON LOCAL HONEY
6 ICE CUBES

1. Pour the almond milk into the blender.

2. Add the banana and process until smooth; then add the figs and honey, blending until the texture is creamy once again.

3. Incorporate the ice cubes, blending and pulsing until smooth. If the mixture is too thick for your liking, add a little more almond milk to thin it out.

4. Pour into a glass and enjoy.

Apple-Cinnamon Power Breakfast

YIELDS 2 CUPS

▶ 158 CALORIES PER CUP

Apples, oats, and cinnamon are a time-honored combination, not only because they taste fantastic together, but also because all of these ingredients are wonderfully healthful. The oats and apples provide fiber and an abundance of vitamins, and the almond milk in this recipe provides protein. Consuming as little as ½ teaspoon of cinnamon daily can lower bad (LDL) cholesterol, plus this warm spice is known as a natural cure for headaches, including tough migraines. Try cinnamon in other smoothie recipes, too.

This recipe is fantastic with extra spices—add ¼ teaspoon of powdered ginger, a pinch of nutmeg, or a pinch of cloves to the cinnamon before tossing it with the apples.

¼ CUP ROLLED OATS

1 CUP UNSWEETENED ALMOND MILK, DIVIDED

2 ORGANIC APPLES, CORED AND CUT INTO 1-INCH CHUNKS

½ TEASPOON CINNAMON

1 TABLESPOON LOCAL HONEY

4 TO 6 ICE CUBES (OPTIONAL)

1. Soak the oats in ½ cup of the unsweetened almond milk; set aside for at least 5 minutes.

2. Pour the remaining ½ cup of almond milk into the blender.

3. Toss the apple chunks with the cinnamon, add them to the blender, and process until smooth.

4. Add the oats and any remaining liquid to the blender along with the honey, then blend until smooth and creamy, adding four to six ice cubes if you prefer an icy texture.

5. Spoon or pour into a glass and enjoy.

Heart-Healthy Fruit and Oat Shake

YIELDS 4 CUPS

▶ 81 CALORIES PER CUP

Strawberries are very high in vitamins, including vitamin C, and contain an abundance of fiber along with many of the minerals and antioxidants your body requires for good health. The chia seeds provide omega-3 fatty acids and protein, while the tangerines provide an additional nutrition boost.

¼ CUP ROLLED OATS
1 CUP UNSWEETENED ALMOND MILK, DIVIDED
2 CUPS FRESH ORGANIC STRAWBERRIES
2 TANGERINES, PEELED AND SEEDED
2 TABLESPOONS CHIA SEEDS, SOAKED IN WATER FOR 20 MINUTES
4 ICE CUBES

1. Soak the oats in ½ cup of the unsweetened almond milk; set aside for at least 5 minutes.

2. Pour the remaining ½ cup of almond milk into the blender. Add the strawberries, tangerines, and soaked chia seeds, then blend and pulse until the mixture is smooth.

3. Add the oats and any remaining almond milk to the blender, processing until they have been thoroughly incorporated.

4. Add the ice cubes; blend and pulse until smooth.

5. Pour into a glass and enjoy.

Nuts over Oatmeal Energy Shake

YIELDS 2 CUPS

▶ 227 CALORIES PER CUP

When you're feeling hungry and unhealthy foods seem to be calling your name, turn to this delicious, protein-rich smoothie. The cashew butter adds extra protein while the fiber-rich oats fill you up. Naturally sweet honey, almond milk, and cinnamon will satisfy you and make you feel fantastic for hours.

¼ CUP ROLLED OATS

1 CUP UNSWEETENED ALMOND MILK, DIVIDED

1 BANANA, PEELED AND CUT INTO 1-INCH CHUNKS

½ TEASPOON CINNAMON

2 TABLESPOONS CASHEW BUTTER

1 TABLESPOON LOCAL HONEY

4 ICE CUBES

1. Soak the oats in ½ cup of the unsweetened almond milk; set aside for at least 5 minutes.

2. Pour the remaining ½ cup of almond milk into the blender.

3. Roll the banana chunks in the cinnamon and add them to the almond milk, then process until smooth.

continued ▶

4. Add the oats and any remaining liquid, along with the cashew butter and honey.

5. Blend and pulse until smooth, adding a small amount of water or additional almond milk to thin the mixture, if desired.

6. Incorporate the ice cubes, pulsing and blending until the desired consistency has been achieved.

7. Pour into a glass and enjoy.

Oat-Berry Breakfast Breeze

YIELDS 3 CUPS

▶ 92 CALORIES PER CUP

Frozen berry blends are easy to keep on hand and are often less expensive than fresh berries. A blend containing strawberries, blackberries, raspberries, and blueberries offers few calories while providing a substantial amount of antioxidants, vitamins, and minerals. Though this breakfast smoothie is lighter than some others in this chapter, it has a substantial amount of fiber as well as some protein, so you'll feel fully satisfied after drinking it.

If you'd like to cut preparation time even further, soak your oats in the refrigerator overnight.

¼ CUP ROLLED OATS
1 CUP UNSWEETENED ALMOND MILK, DIVIDED
2 CUPS FROZEN MIXED BERRIES
STEVIA EXTRACT

1. Soak the oats in ½ cup of the unsweetened almond milk; set aside for at least 5 minutes.

2. Pour the remaining ½ cup of unsweetened almond milk into the blender, add the berries, and blend until smooth.

3. Add the soaked oats and any additional liquid, along with a few drops of stevia extract to taste, if desired. Blend until smooth and creamy.

4. Pour into a glass and enjoy.

Hearty Banana-Flax Power Shake

YIELDS 2 CUPS

▶ 150 CALORIES PER CUP

Flaxseed has been linked to reduced risk of cancer, stroke, heart disease, and diabetes and is an excellent source of healthy omega-3 fatty acid. Add one tablespoon of ground flaxseed to any of your favorite smoothie recipes for numerous nutritional benefits that won't change the flavors.

½ CUP UNSWEETENED ALMOND MILK

1 BANANA, PEELED AND CUT INTO 1-INCH CHUNKS

1 TABLESPOON GROUND FLAXSEED

1 CUP FRESH OR FROZEN BLUEBERRIES

1 TABLESPOON LOCAL HONEY

¼ TEASPOON PURE VANILLA EXTRACT

4 TO 6 ICE CUBES (OPTIONAL)

1. Pour the almond milk into the blender.

2. Toss the banana chunks with the flaxseed, then add them to the blender, pureeing until smooth.

3. Add the blueberries, honey, and vanilla and process until smooth. Add ice cubes if desired, pulsing and blending until the preferred consistency is achieved.

4. Pour into a glass and enjoy.

Fruity Tofu Scramble

YIELDS 4 CUPS

▶ 112 CALORIES PER CUP

Try this high-protein breakfast smoothie instead of cholesterol-laden scrambled eggs. It offers a substantial amount of protein, a smooth and rich consistency, and plenty of delicious fruit flavor. The strawberries and mango provide an abundance of vitamins, antioxidants, and minerals, while the honey and vanilla extract enhance the natural flavors of the fruit. This recipe works just as well with fresh fruit, if preferred, and it's easy to transform the flavor simply by using different types of your favorite fruits.

When shopping for tofu, choose a brand that doesn't contain GMO soy, if possible. While discussions are ongoing as to whether GMO foods are harmful to human health, it's best to err on the side of caution.

1 CUP UNSWEETENED ALMOND MILK

1 BANANA, PEELED AND CUT INTO 1-INCH CHUNKS

4 OUNCES SILKEN TOFU, CUT INTO 1-INCH SQUARES

1 CUP FROZEN STRAWBERRIES

1 CUP FROZEN MANGO CHUNKS

½ TEASPOON PURE VANILLA EXTRACT

1 TABLESPOON LOCAL HONEY

1. Combine the almond milk, banana, and tofu in the blender and process until smooth.

2. Add the strawberries, mango, vanilla, and honey, then process again until all ingredients have been incorporated.

3. Pour into a glass and enjoy.

Breakfast of Champions

YIELDS 2 CUPS

▶ 160 CALORIES PER CUP

Protein powder is formulated for easy digestion, and depending on the brand, it can contain a variety of nutrients that are necessary for good health. This powerfully nutritious breakfast smoothie also contains flaxseed for an omega-3 boost, along with antioxidant-rich dark berries and cranberry juice. It's excellent with frozen cherries instead of berries, and it's also very good with peaches or nectarines.

¼ CUP UNSWEETENED CRANBERRY JUICE

¼ CUP WATER

1 SERVING VANILLA- OR BERRY-FLAVORED PROTEIN POWDER

1 TABLESPOON GROUND FLAXSEED

1 CUP FROZEN MIXED BERRIES

1 TABLESPOON LOCAL HONEY

6 ICE CUBES

1. Pour the cranberry juice and water into the blender, along with the protein powder and flaxseed. Blend well.

2. Add the frozen berries, honey, and ice cubes and blend until all ingredients have been well incorporated. If the mixture is too thick, add water until the desired consistency has been achieved.

3. Pour into a glass and enjoy.

CHAPTER SIX

Smoothies for Health

Smoothies aren't just quick, convenient, and portable—they're also ideal for promoting good health in a way that's fun and delicious. You can incorporate all sorts of healthful ingredients into smoothies, focusing on antioxidants, detoxifiers, minerals, or any other type of nutrient you feel your body is craving. You can even make smoothies that offer a multitude of benefits; in fact, most of the recipes in this chapter—and in the remainder of this book—do just that.

Many of the recipes in this chapter are suggested in the smoothie cleanse menu plans found in Chapter Four, but you can use them any time you like. As with other recipes in this book, they can be modified as you see fit. Consider adding protein powder, superfoods, and other supplements. Though some supplements can alter the flavor slightly, many are not even noticeable. Chia seeds, hemp seeds, ground flaxseed, and aloe vera juice are a few excellent additives with very mild flavors.

Whether you're hoping to stave off rapid aging or ward off disease by increasing your antioxidant intake, boost your immunity with an abundance of vitamins, or accomplish any other health-related goal, you can use smoothies to ensure that you receive the best natural nutrition possible. After all, when you consume the best foods nature has to offer, you benefit in many ways, both physically and mentally.

Eat a variety of fresh foods for good health—While it's possible to take a vitamin supplement to promote good health, it's also important to consume a diet that contains a wide variety of whole, unadulterated foods. Doing so will greatly increase the likelihood that you will take in sufficient quantities of all the nutrients your body needs, and it may help to prevent illness, including cancer, diabetes, and cardiovascular disease.

Pomegranate Protection

YIELDS 3 CUPS

▶ 118 CALORIES PER CUP

Pomegranates are packed with antioxidants, plus they offer refreshing flavor. It can be tough to seed and juice a pomegranate, so purchase pure pomegranate juice at the market if you need to—a little bit of this delicious nectar goes a long way. The grapes, frozen berries, and dried goji berries in this recipe offer numerous antioxidants, too, so enjoy this delightful smoothie knowing that you're protecting your body from dangerous toxins. This recipe works very well with any type of fresh or frozen berries, so feel free to use whatever is in season or on sale.

½ CUP PURE POMEGRANATE JUICE
½ CUP PURPLE SEEDLESS GRAPES
1 CUP FROZEN MIXED BERRIES
¼ CUP DRIED GOJI BERRIES
2 TABLESPOONS CHIA SEEDS, SOAKED IN WATER FOR
    20 MINUTES
6 ICE CUBES

1. Combine the pomegranate juice and grapes in the blender and process until smooth.

2. Add the frozen berries, dried goji berries, and soaked chia seeds, then pulse and blend until smooth.

3. Incorporate the ice cubes, pulsing and blending until the desired consistency has been achieved.

4. Pour into a glass and enjoy.

Filling Avocado Freeze

YIELDS 4 CUPS

▶ 106 CALORIES PER CUP

Avocados are an excellent source of healthy plant-based fat, which our bodies need for maintaining healthy skin, hair, and tissues. The acai juice and dark berries in this smoothie contain high levels of antioxidants, which are important for heart health and longevity, and the yogurt contains protein to keep you feeling full for an extended period of time. Incorporate your favorite superfood to give this recipe a customizable boost of nutrition. If blackberries aren't available, try using an equal amount of blueberries, raspberries, or any of your favorite fruits instead.

½ CUP ACAI JUICE
1 CUP GREEK YOGURT OR NON-DAIRY YOGURT
¼ RIPE AVOCADO, PEELED AND PITTED
2 CUPS BLACKBERRIES, FRESH OR FROZEN
6 ICE CUBES
LOCAL HONEY OR STEVIA EXTRACT (OPTIONAL)

1. Combine the acai juice, yogurt, and avocado in the blender, processing until smooth.

2. Add the blackberries and ice cubes, then pulse and blend until fully incorporated.

3. If the smoothie is too tart for your taste, blend in a tablespoon of honey or a few drops of stevia extract for natural sweetness.

4. Pour into a glass and enjoy.

Happy Heart

YIELDS 4 CUPS

▶ 91 CALORIES PER CUP

Vitamin C is a powerful antioxidant, and it's also excellent for the circulatory system. It helps to reduce the potential for blood vessel damage, plus it helps boost collagen production, which is essential for building healthy veins and arteries. This fantastic smoothie contains an abundance of vitamin C, along with vitamins E and A, which are also essential to heart health. To make this smoothie into a satisfying meal replacement shake, simply add a scoop of your favorite vanilla- or berry-flavored protein powder. You may need to add a little more water or orange juice if you modify the recipe this way.

1 CUP FRESHLY SQUEEZED ORANGE JUICE
1 BANANA, PEELED AND CUT INTO 1-INCH CHUNKS
1 CUP ORGANIC STRAWBERRIES, CLEANED AND HALVED
¼ RIPE AVOCADO, PEELED AND PITTED
1 CUP FRESH CANTALOUPE CHUNKS
6 ICE CUBES

1. Combine the orange juice and banana in the blender, processing until smooth.

2. Add the strawberries, avocado, and cantaloupe, blending again until all ingredients have been incorporated.

3. Add the ice cubes, then blend and pulse until the desired consistency has been achieved.

4. Pour into a glass and enjoy.

Chocolate-Cherry Champion

YIELDS 4 CUPS

▶ 119 CALORIES PER CUP

Chocolate isn't just one of the world's favorite foods—it's also amazingly healthy, with many of the same benefits attributed to other dark-colored fruits such as blueberries and blackberries. Ounce for ounce, pure chocolate contains almost eight times as many antioxidants as strawberries, along with important nutrients that help to reduce blood pressure and keep LDL cholesterol in check. It also contains a little healthy monounsaturated fat, which can help keep you feeling satisfied and doing your best work for an extended period of time.

1 CUP UNSWEETENED ALMOND MILK

1 BANANA, PEELED AND CUT INTO 1-INCH CHUNKS

2 TABLESPOONS PURE UNSWEETENED COCOA POWDER

1 SCOOP CHOCOLATE-FLAVORED PROTEIN POWDER

2 CUPS FROZEN SWEET CHERRIES

1. Pour the almond milk into the blender.

2. Roll the banana chunks in the cocoa powder and add them to the almond milk along with the protein powder.

3. Blend until smooth, then add the cherries, blending and pulsing until all ingredients are well incorporated.

4. Spoon or pour into a glass and enjoy.

Blueberry-Avocado Body Bliss

YIELDS 4 CUPS

▶ 107 CALORIES PER CUP

Healthy skin, shiny hair, and strong nails begin with good nutrition. Brimming with avocado, blueberries, and other delicious ingredients, this recipe offers protein, fiber, antioxidants, and healthy monounsaturated fat, along with many essential vitamins and minerals.

Add a few drops of stevia extract for extra sweetness if needed, and feel free to experiment with different flavors by replacing the blueberries with two cups of your favorite fresh or frozen fruit.

½ CUP UNSWEETENED ALMOND MILK

½ CUP GREEK YOGURT OR NON-DAIRY YOGURT

1 BANANA, PEELED AND CUT INTO 1-INCH CHUNKS

¼ RIPE AVOCADO, PEELED AND PITTED

2 CUPS FRESH OR FROZEN BLUEBERRIES

¼ TEASPOON PURE VANILLA EXTRACT

6 ICE CUBES

1. Combine the almond milk, yogurt, banana, and avocado in the blender and process until the mixture is smooth.

2. Add the blueberries, vanilla, and ice cubes, blending and pulsing until all ingredients have been thoroughly incorporated.

3. Spoon or pour into a glass and enjoy.

Purple Grape–Papaya Protection

YIELDS 4 CUPS

▶ 54 CALORIES PER CUP

Protect your eyes, internal organs, and immunity with this delicious yet surprisingly low-calorie smoothie. Grapes contain high levels of vitamins A, C, and B-6 and are linked to the prevention of cataracts, macular degeneration, kidney disorders, and other ailments. They also contain flavonoids and micronutrients including copper, manganese, and iron, which are important for maintaining strong, healthy bones. Papayas have many of the same essential nutrients, along with important enzymes that aid the digestive process.

If you prefer a very thick, icy smoothie, freeze the grapes and papaya beforehand.

1 CUP PURE ACAI JUICE
2 CUPS PURPLE GRAPES
1 CUP FRESH PAPAYA CHUNKS
6 ICE CUBES

1. Combine the acai juice and grapes in the blender and process until smooth.

2. Add the papaya, processing until smooth.

3. Incorporate the ice cubes, blending until the desired consistency has been achieved.

4. Pour into a glass and enjoy.

Ravishing Raspberry Ripple

YIELDS 4 CUPS

▶ 80 CALORIES PER CUP

Beauty begins on the inside, and this luscious but healthful smoothie can help you achieve it. Low in calories, but high in fiber and antioxidants such as vitamin C, raspberries have plenty of essential minerals including potassium, iron, copper, and manganese. In addition, they contain vitamin K and B-complex vitamins, all of which are vital to maintaining a healthy metabolism and the assimilation of protein, carbohydrates, and fat.

You can make this recipe even healthier by adding powdered camu camu berry, a handful of dried goji berries, or a tablespoon of local bee pollen. If no raspberries are available, feel free to substitute another fruit—blueberries, blackberries, and cherries are all excellent options.

½ CUP UNSWEETENED ALMOND MILK

½ CUP GREEK YOGURT OR NON-DAIRY YOGURT

1 BANANA, PEELED AND CUT INTO 1-INCH CHUNKS

2 CUPS FRESH OR FROZEN RASPBERRIES

¼ TEASPOON PURE VANILLA EXTRACT

6 ICE CUBES

continued ▶

Ravishing Raspberry Ripple   *continued* ▶

1. Combine the almond milk, yogurt, and banana in the blender and process until smooth.

2. Add the raspberries, vanilla, and ice cubes, pulsing and blending until thoroughly incorporated.

3. Spoon or pour into a glass and enjoy.

Coconut Craving

▶ 270 CALORIES PER CUP

Coconut is rich in lauric acid, a powerful immunity booster. In addition, it contains high levels of protein, fiber, and fat to quell hunger pangs. This hearty meal replacement smoothie is higher in calories than most of the others in this book, but it can help you beat unhealthy cravings and keep you on track, particularly if you're undertaking a smoothie cleanse.

½ CUP COCONUT WATER
1 BANANA, PEELED AND CUT INTO 1-INCH CHUNKS
1 CUP SHREDDED UNSWEETENED COCONUT
1 SCOOP VANILLA-FLAVORED PROTEIN POWDER
¼ TEASPOON PURE VANILLA EXTRACT
6 ICE CUBES
STEVIA EXTRACT (OPTIONAL)

1. Combine the coconut water and banana in the blender and process until smooth.

2. Add the coconut, protein powder, and vanilla, blending and pulsing until smooth.

3. Incorporate the ice cubes, continuing to blend until the desired consistency has been achieved.

4. Add a few drops of stevia extract if the smoothie isn't sweet enough for you.

5. Pour into a glass and enjoy.

Tofu Temptation

▶ 106 CALORIES PER CUP

Tofu is an excellent source of protein, calcium, vitamins, and minerals, making it a great substitute for animal products. Pineapple and mango provide an abundance of nutrients, including important enzymes that aid in healthy digestion. This filling smoothie makes the perfect anti-dote to cravings for foods that harm the body when eaten in excess.

This recipe works very well with frozen pineapple and mango chunks; you can also pre-freeze your banana chunks for an even more decadent tasting treat.

When shopping for tofu, choose a brand that doesn't contain GMO soy, if possible. While discussions are ongoing as to whether GMO foods are harmful to human health, it's best to err on the side of caution.

½ CUP FRESHLY SQUEEZED ORANGE JUICE

4 OUNCES SILKEN TOFU

1 BANANA, PEELED AND CUT INTO 1-INCH CHUNKS

1 CUP FRESH PINEAPPLE CHUNKS

1 CUP FRESH MANGO CHUNKS

¼ TEASPOON PURE VANILLA EXTRACT

6 ICE CUBES

1. Combine the orange juice, tofu, and banana in the blender and process until smooth.

2. Add the pineapple and mango, blending and pulsing until incorporated, then add the vanilla and ice cubes, continuing to blend until the desired consistency has been achieved.

3. Spoon or pour into a glass and enjoy.

Acai Anti-Aging Shake

YIELDS 4 CUPS

▶ 68 CALORIES PER CUP

Dark-colored fruits, including acai berries, are inextricably linked with youthful good health, as they contain high levels of important antioxidants that help ward off damage caused by exposure to everyday toxins found in the food we eat, the water we drink, the air we breathe, and the chemicals to which we are exposed. Not only is this low-calorie purple smoothie a beautiful treat for the eyes, but it also tastes delicious.

For a delightful icy treat, use frozen berries and grapes rather than fresh ones. You may need to use more acai juice or a little water if you do this, since freezing almost all of your smoothie ingredients yields a much thicker beverage.

1 CUP PURE ACAI JUICE
1 CUP FRESH BLUEBERRIES
1 CUP FRESH BLACKBERRIES
1 CUP PURPLE GRAPES
6 ICE CUBES

1. Combine the acai juice, blueberries, and blackberries in the blender, alternately blending and pulsing until smooth.

2. Add the grapes to the blender, alternately blending and pulsing until smooth.

3. Add the ice cubes, blending and pulsing until they have been thoroughly incorporated and the desired consistency has been achieved.

4. Pour into a glass and enjoy.

CHAPTER SEVEN

Smoothies for Weight Loss

Smoothies are the perfect food for weight loss, whether you consume them instead of commercially produced meal replacement shakes or in place of unhealthy meals and snacks you may be eating now.

Many of the smoothies in this chapter are not only low in calories, but also nutritionally dense—something that cannot be said of many processed foods meant to be eaten for weight loss. In addition to important vitamins, minerals, and micronutrients, the fruits and vegetables in these smoothies contain high levels of water, which is vital to healthy weight loss. They contain fiber, too, which helps you feel full, so you won't wind up hungrily consuming foods that do nothing to help you meet your goals.

When drinking smoothies as part of a healthy weight loss plan, pay close attention to the foods you're eating at other meals. Focus on plant-based nutrition, eliminate sources of unhealthy fat and cholesterol, and stop eating sugary snacks and processed foods that contain hidden sugar in the form of high fructose corn syrup. At the same time, find ways to make old favorites healthier so you don't feel deprived. Keep drinking smoothies after you've lost weight, and you'll find that it's easy to keep unwanted pounds from making their way back to you.

Finally, be sure to exercise most days. As little as fifteen to thirty minutes of movement will make a huge difference if you're sedentary now—and with smoothies powering your life, you'll very likely discover that you have a strong desire to make exercise part of each day.

These recipes are easy to make and are delicious, too. Feel free to use substitutions if you like. You can transform any low-calorie smoothie recipe into a simple, nutritious meal by adding your favorite protein powder.

Increase weight loss success by journaling—*Many people who have successfully lost weight and who have kept that weight off have something in common—they tracked their food intake during the weight loss process. Keeping a simple food journal that details what you ate, when you ate it, and how you were feeling at the time you ate can be an enlightening process that clues you in to habits that can derail weight loss. All you need is a notebook and something to write with; if you prefer to use electronics, you'll find that there are many free food tracking applications available for computers and smartphones alike.*

Slender Sensation

YIELDS 4 CUPS

▶ 20 CALORIES PER CUP

This refreshing low-calorie smoothie contains green tea, which has been linked to healthy weight loss. The strawberries add vitamin C, as well as important phytochemicals, B-complex vitamins, and plenty of minerals including copper, iodine, and iron.

Give this smoothie a boost by incorporating a little of your favorite superfood. For a treat that's even icier, freeze your green tea in an ice cube tray before preparing the recipe.

1 CUP CHILLED GREEN TEA
½ LEMON, PEELED AND SEEDED
2 CUPS FRESH OR FROZEN STRAWBERRIES
8 ICE CUBES
STEVIA EXTRACT

1. Pour the tea into the blender.

2. Add the lemon and strawberries, blending until smooth.

3. Add the ice cubes and stevia to taste, blending and pulsing until the desired consistency has been achieved.

4. Spoon or pour into a glass and enjoy.

Melon-Mint Refresher

YIELDS 4 CUPS

▶ 32 CALORIES PER CUP

This delightful smoothie has a clean, fresh taste and just the right amount of natural sweetness, along with vitamins, minerals, and fiber. Perfect for cooling off after a workout and equally nice while relaxing with friends, this smoothie is very easy to make, particularly if you prepare the ingredients in advance.

For an even more refreshing flavor, add a small handful of fresh mint leaves along with the ice cubes.

1 CUP CHILLED PEPPERMINT TEA
2 CUPS FRESH HONEYDEW MELON CHUNKS
STEVIA EXTRACT (OPTIONAL)
8 ICE CUBES

1. Combine the tea and honeydew in the blender and process until smooth.

2. Add stevia to taste, if desired.

3. Add the ice cubes, then pulse and blend until the desired consistency has been achieved.

4. Spoon or pour into a glass and enjoy.

Watermelon Wellness

YIELDS 4 CUPS

▶ 20 CALORIES PER CUP

Though low in calories, this luscious smoothie offers plenty of watermelon flavor, plus nutrients including lycopene, potassium, and beta carotene. Use either seeded or seedless watermelon; the seeds will be completely pulverized during the blending process and will add a bit of satisfying protein and fiber without altering the flavor.

To make this summertime recipe frostier, freeze the watermelon chunks ahead of time.

1 CUP CHILLED GREEN TEA
2 CUPS CHILLED FRESH WATERMELON CHUNKS
8 ICE CUBES

1. Combine the tea and watermelon in the blender and process until smooth.

2. Add the ice cubes, then pulse and blend until the desired consistency has been achieved.

3. Spoon or pour into a glass and enjoy.

Greek Protein Punch

YIELDS 4 CUPS

▶ 87 CALORIES PER CUP

Here's a wonderful meal replacement smoothie with plenty of protein, just a little healthful fat, and an abundance of fiber. This recipe aids in digestion by incorporating yogurt, which contains probiotics. Choose yogurt with live cultures to ensure that you receive all of the health benefits.

½ CUP UNSWEETENED ALMOND MILK
½ CUP NONFAT GREEK OR NONDAIRY YOGURT
1 BANANA, PEELED AND CUT INTO 1-INCH CHUNKS
1 CUP FRESH OR FROZEN PINEAPPLE CHUNKS
1 CUP FRESH OR FROZEN RASPBERRIES
4 ICE CUBES

1. Combine the almond milk, yogurt, and banana in the blender and process until smooth.

2. Add the pineapple and raspberries, blending until well incorporated.

3. Add the ice cubes, pulsing and blending until the desired consistency has been achieved. Add more ice cubes for a thicker, more hydrating smoothie.

4. Spoon or pour into a glass and enjoy.

Mindful Melon

YIELDS 5 CUPS

▶ 88 CALORIES PER CUP

A scrumptious meal replacement smoothie with a light, refreshing taste, this recipe uses almond milk and yogurt for protein, chia seeds for omega-3 fatty acid, and a delicious blend of melon and mango for unbeatable flavor, healthy fiber, and lots of essential vitamins and minerals.

This recipe can be modified to include any of your favorite fruits; try experimenting with various combinations such as peaches and cherries, apricots and pineapple, or apples and blueberries.

½ CUP UNSWEETENED ALMOND MILK
1 CUP NONFAT GREEK YOGURT OR NONDAIRY YOGURT
2 CUPS FRESH CANTALOUPE CHUNKS
1 CUP FRESH MANGO CHUNKS
2 TABLESPOONS CHIA SEEDS, SOAKED FOR 20 MINUTES
8 ICE CUBES

1. Combine the almond milk, yogurt, cantaloupe, and mango in the blender and process until smooth.

2. Add the chia seeds and ice cubes, blending and pulsing until they have been thoroughly incorporated.

3. Spoon or pour into a glass and enjoy.

Banana-Avocado Tummy Tamer

YIELDS 3 CUPS

▶ 118 CALORIES PER CUP

This smoothie is a very satisfying meal replacement shake since it provides protein, fiber, a little bit of healthy fat, and plenty of flavor; add your favorite superfood to give it even more nutritional power. Bananas offer potassium, while papayas contain an enzyme called papain. Both of these nutrients help to calm the digestive system and ease bloating. The avocado is a helpful boost that slows sugar absorption to keep you feeling full.

½ CUP UNSWEETENED ALMOND MILK
½ CUP NONFAT GREEK YOGURT OR NONDAIRY YOGURT
1 BANANA, PEELED AND CUT INTO 1-INCH CHUNKS
1 CUP FRESH PAPAYA CHUNKS
¼ RIPE AVOCADO, PEELED AND PITTED
1 TABLESPOON GROUND FLAXSEED
4 ICE CUBES

1. Combine the almond milk, yogurt, banana, papaya, avocado, and flaxseed in the blender and process until smooth.

2. Add the ice cubes, pulsing and blending until the desired consistency is achieved. If your smoothie is too thick, add a little water or almond milk.

3. Spoon or pour into a glass and enjoy.

Mango Enlightenment

YIELDS 3 CUPS

▶ 30 CALORIES PER CUP

Ultra-low in calories yet wonderfully nutritious, this juicy smoothie contains fiber, vitamin C, beta carotene, and potassium, courtesy of the mango. These essential nutrients promote nervous system health while protecting the immune system and reducing the potential for heart disease.

It's easy to transform this smoothie into a meal replacement shake by replacing the tea with unsweetened almond milk and adding a scoop of your favorite protein powder.

1 CUP CHILLED PEACH-FLAVORED HERBAL TEA
1 CUP FRESH MANGO CHUNKS
¼ TEASPOON PURE VANILLA EXTRACT
8 ICE CUBES

1. Combine the tea and mango in the blender and process until smooth.

2. Add the vanilla and ice cubes, then blend and pulse until the desired consistency has been achieved.

3. Pour into a glass and enjoy.

Kiwi-Banana Belly Blaster

YIELDS 4 CUPS

▶ 150 CALORIES PER CUP

Although this tasty meal replacement smoothie will leave you feeling satisfied, it contains no guilt-inducing ingredients and offers superior nutrition. Kiwi fruit are rich in vitamins including C and E, and they contain high levels of potassium, essential fatty acids, and enzymes. The avocado, protein powder, and banana keep you feeling full so you can keep annoying cravings at bay.

You can make this lovely light-green smoothie even more nutritious by adding a handful of fresh leafy greens or a bit of powdered chlorella, blue-green algae, or spirulina.

1 CUP UNSWEETENED ALMOND MILK
1 BANANA, PEELED AND CUT INTO 1-INCH CHUNKS
1 SCOOP VANILLA- OR BERRY-FLAVORED PROTEIN POWDER
¼ RIPE AVOCADO, PEELED AND PITTED
4 KIWI FRUIT, PEELED AND HALVED
1 CUP FROZEN GREEN GRAPES

1. Combine the almond milk, banana, protein powder, and avocado in the blender, processing until smooth.

2. Add the kiwi and grapes, then pulse and blend until all ingredients have been completely incorporated.

3. Pour into a glass and enjoy.

Purple Perfection

YIELDS 5 CUPS

▶ 44 CALORIES PER CUP

Eliminate cravings for unhealthy snacks with this low-calorie smoothie that can satisfy your sweet tooth while giving you a dose of healthy hydration. In addition, you'll receive an abundance of antioxidants, flavonoids, and vitamins, thanks to the blackberries that give this tasty treat its appealing purple hue.

This recipe works well with any berries you happen to have on hand, including fresh or frozen berry blends, raspberries, strawberries, or boysenberries. For an icier smoothie, freeze the tea before you get started.

1 CUP CHILLED BERRY-FLAVORED HERBAL TEA
2 CUPS BLACKBERRIES
1 CUP BLUEBERRIES
8 ICE CUBES
STEVIA EXTRACT (OPTIONAL)

1. Combine the tea and blackberries in the blender and process until smooth.

2. Add the blueberries and the ice cubes, pulsing and blending until they have been well incorporated.

3. Add a few drops of stevia if your smoothie isn't sweet enough.

4. Spoon or pour into a glass and enjoy.

Mango Miracle

YIELDS 4 CUPS

▶ 107 CALORIES PER CUP

Brimming with vitamins A and C, this filling meal replacement smoothie combines sweet, tangy mangos and mild-tasting cashew butter, which will keep you feeling satisfied for hours thanks to the fiber, protein, and healthy fat it contains. Great any time of day, this smoothie holds up well in a travel mug and is perfect for lunch on the go.

1 CUP UNSWEETENED ALMOND MILK
1 BANANA, PEELED AND CUT INTO 1-INCH CHUNKS
2 TABLESPOONS CASHEW BUTTER
2 CUPS FRESH OR FROZEN MANGO CHUNKS

1. Combine the almond milk, banana, and cashew butter in the blender, processing until smooth.

2. Add the mango, pulsing and blending until well incorporated.

3. This is a very thick smoothie; you may need to add a little more almond milk or some filtered water if the blender's blades start to stick.

4. Spoon or pour into a glass and enjoy.

CHAPTER EIGHT

Green Smoothies

Green smoothies are more popular than ever, and that's not at all surprising since they offer delicious flavor and superior nutrition. As a rule, green smoothies contain vegetables as well as fruits. While some find this concept to be slightly strange, there are many vegetables with mild flavors that are often completely masked by the stronger flavors of fruits and other ingredients.

A green smoothie can be sweet or savory, tangy or spicy. The flavor combinations you can create are endless—and even if you're among those who wonder whether these odd-looking blends really are edible, you'll soon find yourself wishing that you had discovered them sooner.

When making green smoothies, be certain that you wash your leafy greens very well since bits of sandy soil sometimes cling to them. After washing, chop them roughly before measuring. This breaks up long fibers and makes the leaves easier for your blender to handle. Finally, if you decide that you love green smoothies and want to drink them frequently, be sure to use a variety of different greens to ensure that you're providing yourself with a wide range of nutrients. This is especially important if you are cleansing.

The recipes in this chapter are meant to introduce you to green smoothies with an interesting variety of blends that will help you ease your way into trying even more adventurous combinations in the future. If you feel the urge to make new green smoothie creations, simply try adding your favorite greens to any of the recipes in this book. While you might occasionally blunder, you will almost certainly create new healthful favorites.

Store greens properly to prevent spoilage—*Greens can go bad quickly–and you can often taste or smell spoilage occurring before it is visible. Since spoiled greens can make you sick, it's important to use only the freshest greens in your smoothies. Keep those leafy green vegetables fresh by removing them from the container they came in, drying them well, and then placing them back into the container with a few folded paper towels underneath to keep dampness at bay. Only purchase the amount of greens you will be able to use within a few days, and you'll never have to deal with spoilage.*

Green Grape Greatness

YIELDS 5 CUPS

▶ 49 CALORIES PER CUP

If you're looking for an easy introduction to green smoothies, this recipe will win you over in a flash. Grapes offer many nutrients, and the fiber they contain prevents the natural sugar from being metabolized by the body too quickly. Baby spinach has a mild taste that is often difficult to detect in smoothies, particularly when fruit takes center stage.

To transform the flavor of this recipe, replace the grapes with a different fruit. Mangos, peaches, and pineapple are all perfect candidates.

1 CUP CHILLED GREEN TEA
1 BANANA, PEELED AND CUT INTO 1-INCH CHUNKS
2 CUPS SEEDLESS GREEN GRAPES
JUICE FROM ¼ LEMON
1 CUP CHOPPED BABY SPINACH, LOOSELY PACKED
8 ICE CUBES

1. Combine the tea and banana in the blender, processing until smooth.

2. Add the grapes, lemon juice, and spinach, and process until well incorporated.

3. Add the ice cubes, blending and pulsing until the desired consistency has been achieved.

4. Pour into a glass and enjoy.

Protective Peaches and Greens

YIELDS 4 CUPS

▶ 71 CALORIES PER CUP

This simple recipe has a funny green color, but don't let that fool you—it tastes absolutely fantastic. Leafy greens provide numerous antioxidants, vitamins, and minerals that protect the body's cells from damage. Peaches also contain many essential nutrients along with a sweet, juicy flavor that's difficult to resist.

Make this smoothie into a meal replacement shake by adding one scoop of your favorite vanilla-flavored protein powder to the blender along with the peaches and lettuce.

1 CUP CHILLED PEACH-FLAVORED HERBAL TEA
1 BANANA, PEELED AND CUT INTO 1-INCH CHUNKS
4 RIPE PEACHES, PITTED AND CUT INTO 1-INCH CHUNKS
2 CUPS CHOPPED ROMAINE LETTUCE, LOOSELY PACKED
¼ TEASPOON PURE VANILLA EXTRACT
8 ICE CUBES

1. Combine the tea and banana in the blender, processing until smooth.

2. Add the peaches, lettuce, and vanilla, and blend until fully incorporated.

3. Add the ice cubes, blending and pulsing until the desired consistency has been achieved.

4. Pour into a glass and enjoy.

Green Love Machine

▶ 77 CALORIES PER CUP

One way that fruits and vegetables enhance wellness is by improving our ability to enjoy a healthy love life. All leafy greens contain folate, fiber, and magnesium, which are essential for maintaining a healthy reproductive system. In addition, treating your body and brain to optimum nutrition from natural sources is a great way to ensure that you look and feel your best—two things that can help improve all aspects of life, including intimacy.

If you decide to add protein to this smoothie, use protein powder or nut milk, as the high concentration of citrus in this recipe can cause dairy and soy milk to curdle.

1 CUP CHILLED CITRUS-FLAVORED HERBAL TEA

1 BANANA, PEELED AND CUT INTO 1-INCH CHUNKS

1 ORANGE, PEELED, SEEDED, AND SEPARATED INTO SEGMENTS

2 TANGERINES, PEELED, SEEDED, AND SEPARATED
    INTO SEGMENTS

2 KIWI FRUIT, PEELED AND HALVED

1 CUP CHOPPED BABY BOK CHOY LEAVES, LOOSELY PACKED

8 ICE CUBES

1. Combine the tea and banana in the blender and process until smooth.

2. Add the orange and tangerines, blending until smooth.

continued ▶

Green Love Machine *continued* ▶

3. Add the kiwi and baby bok choy leaves, blending and pulsing until fully incorporated.

4. Add the ice cubes, pulsing and blending until the desired consistency has been achieved.

5. Spoon or pour into a glass and enjoy.

Cucumber-Celery Power Cleanse

YIELDS 4 CUPS

▶ 32 CALORIES PER CUP

Celery contains a lot of water, plenty of minerals, and very few calories, while cucumber is a mild diuretic that can help promote cleansing. Both of these green vegetables are low in calories, as are zucchini, romaine lettuce, and parsley, so you can drink as much of this smoothie as you like without worry.

If you like the flavor of hot spices, pep things up by adding a dash of your favorite hot sauce to your glass and stirring it in before drinking.

1 CUP CHILLED FILTERED WATER

1 LARGE ORGANIC CUCUMBER, PEEL ON, CUT INTO
   1-INCH SEGMENTS

4 STALKS ORGANIC CELERY, LONG FIBROUS STRANDS
   REMOVED, ROUGHLY CHOPPED

1 THREE-INCH PIECE ORGANIC ZUCCHINI, PEEL ON, CUT
   INTO 1-INCH SEGMENTS

2 CUPS CHOPPED ROMAINE LETTUCE, LOOSELY PACKED

¼ CUP FRESH PARSLEY LEAVES, LOOSELY PACKED

JUICE FROM ¼ LEMON

8 ICE CUBES

continued ▶

Cucumber-Celery Power Cleanse *continued* ▶

1. Combine the water, cucumber, celery, and zucchini in blender, processing until smooth.

2. Add the romaine lettuce and parsley, pulsing and blending until fully incorporated.

3. Add the lemon juice and ice cubes, pulsing and blending until the desired consistency has been achieved.

4. Pour into a glass and enjoy.

Melon Mind Meld

YIELDS 4 CUPS

▶ 105 CALORIES PER CUP

The chia seeds in this recipe contain the essential fatty acids your brain needs for optimum function, and the mango contains carotenoids, which protect the nervous system and brain from damage while helping to keep heart disease and high cholesterol at bay. This smoothie is very good for you, and it has a decadent flavor you're certain to love.

1 CUP CHILLED GREEN TEA
1 BANANA, PEELED AND CUT INTO 1-INCH CHUNKS
2 CUPS FRESH OR FROZEN MANGO CHUNKS
2 TABLESPOONS CHIA SEEDS, SOAKED FOR 20 MINUTES
3 APRICOTS, PITTED AND HALVED
2 CUPS CHOPPED BUTTER LETTUCE, LOOSELY PACKED
4 ICE CUBES

1. Pour the tea into the blender and add the banana, processing until smooth.

2. Add the mango, chia seeds, and apricots, then pulse and blend until smooth.

3. Finally, add the butter lettuce and the ice cubes, pulsing and blending until the desired consistency has been achieved.

4. Pour into a glass and enjoy.

Gorgeous Green Machine

YIELDS 6 CUPS

▶ 41 CALORIES PER CUP

Spinach is one of the best foods for skin health, with plenty of vitamins A, E, and C. It contains folate to help improve skin clarity, and the antioxidants aid in promoting healthy cell turnover and repairing past damage.

This smoothie can be easily transformed by substituting various types of fruit in place of some or all of the berries. Try oranges and tangerines with strawberries; papaya and mango with blueberries; or pineapple, mango, and apricot with green tea, spinach, and ice cubes. You'll be amazed at the flavors that emerge when you experiment.

1 CUP CHILLED GREEN TEA
2 CUPS FRESH OR FROZEN STRAWBERRIES
1 CUP FRESH OR FROZEN BLUEBERRIES
1 CUP FRESH OR FROZEN BLACKBERRIES
3 CUPS CHOPPED BABY SPINACH, LOOSELY PACKED
8 ICE CUBES

1. Combine the tea and strawberries in the blender, processing until smooth.

2. Add the blueberries, blackberries, and spinach, blending and pulsing until fully incorporated.

3. Add the ice cubes, blending and pulsing until the desired consistency has been achieved.

4. Spoon or pour into a glass and enjoy.

Veggie Power

▶ 55 CALORIES PER CUP

Savor the taste of summer's fresh vegetables in this recipe. Bell peppers have a mild, slightly sweet flavor that pairs well with fresh herbs and greens. Low in calories yet loaded with essential minerals, vitamins, and phytonutrients, they play a starring role in this delicious all-vegetable smoothie.

1 CUP CHILLED FILTERED WATER

2 GREEN BELL PEPPERS, SEEDED AND CUT INTO 1-INCH CHUNKS

2 YELLOW BELL PEPPERS, SEEDED AND CUT INTO 1-INCH CHUNKS

1 SMALL ORGANIC CUCUMBER, PEEL ON, CUT INTO 1-INCH SEGMENTS

1 GARLIC CLOVE, PEELED AND ROUGHLY CHOPPED

¼ CUP FRESH BASIL LEAVES

JUICE FROM ¼ LEMON

1 CUP CHOPPED BABY KALE, LOOSELY PACKED

4 ICE CUBES

1. Combine the water, bell peppers, cucumber, and garlic in the blender, processing until smooth.

2. Add the basil, lemon juice, and kale, processing again until all ingredients have been completely incorporated.

3. Add the ice cubes, blending and pulsing until the desired consistency has been achieved.

4. Pour into a glass and enjoy.

Green Coconut Colada

▶ 154 CALORIES PER CUP

When you're in the mood for a tropical treat, look no further than this delicious green smoothie. It's got pineapple, coconut, and mango for sweet flavor and balanced nutrition, and it also includes romaine lettuce, which is among the lightest-tasting greens available. If you're hoping to convince a friend or loved one that green smoothies are fantastic, this recipe will help you make your case.

If you don't feel like adding mango, simply increase the amount of pineapple to 3 cups.

1 CUP CHILLED COCONUT WATER
1 BANANA, PEELED AND CUT INTO 1-INCH CHUNKS
2 CUPS FRESH OR FROZEN PINEAPPLE CHUNKS
1 CUP FRESH OR FROZEN MANGO CHUNKS
1 CUP SHREDDED UNSWEETENED COCONUT
2 CUPS CHOPPED ROMAINE LETTUCE, LOOSELY PACKED
8 ICE CUBES

1. Combine the coconut water and banana, blending until smooth.

2. Add the pineapple, mango, and coconut to the blender, processing until well incorporated.

3. Add the romaine and ice cubes, blending and pulsing until the desired consistency has been achieved.

4. Pour into a glass and enjoy.

Spiced Apple

YIELDS 3 CUPS

▶ 58 CALORIES PER CUP

Fresh organic apples are easy to obtain throughout the year in most places, and high-protein alfalfa sprouts are simple to grow in a sunny window, no matter what the season. This tart green smoothie offers satisfying flavors that can tame cravings, yet contains an abundance of essential vitamins, minerals, and antioxidants.

To transform this recipe into a heart-healthy breakfast smoothie, soak ¼ cup of rolled oats in ½ cup of unsweetened almond milk, set aside for at least five minutes, then add to the blender with the sprouts and ice cubes.

2 ORGANIC GRANNY SMITH APPLES, CORED AND CUT INTO
   1-INCH CHUNKS
¼ TEASPOON CINNAMON
1 CUP CHILLED CHAI SPICE TEA
¼ TEASPOON PURE VANILLA EXTRACT
½ CUP ALFALFA SPROUTS
4 ICE CUBES

1. Roll the apple chunks in the cinnamon and add them to the blender along with the tea.

2. Blend until smooth, then add vanilla, alfalfa sprouts, and ice cubes, processing until all ingredients have been well incorporated and the desired consistency has been achieved.

3. Spoon or pour into a glass and enjoy.

Mango Spinach Splash

YIELDS 4 CUPS

▶ 118 CALORIES PER CUP

This luscious smoothie contains an abundance of greens, but don't let that frighten you—it also features four servings of fruit, which provide more than enough sweet-tart flavor to keep the taste of the greens from being overly prominent. Some nutrients found in this smoothie include vitamins C and A, potassium, lutein, folate, and vitamin K, along with plenty of antioxidants.

1 CUP CHILLED CITRUS-FLAVORED GREEN TEA

1 BANANA, PEELED AND CUT INTO 1-INCH CHUNKS

2 CUPS FRESH OR FROZEN MANGO CHUNKS

1 CUP FRESH OR FROZEN PINEAPPLE CHUNKS

1 CUP CHOPPED BABY SPINACH, LOOSELY PACKED

2 CUPS CHOPPED ROMAINE LETTUCE, LOOSELY PACKED

8 ICE CUBES

1. Combine the tea and banana in the blender and process until smooth.

2. Add the mango and pineapple, process until the mixture is smooth once again, and add the spinach and romaine, pulsing and blending until well incorporated.

3. Finally, add the ice cubes, continuing to pulse and blend until the desired texture has been achieved.

4. Pour into a glass and enjoy.

CHAPTER NINE

Energy Boosters

Whether you're facing a long day at work, a challenging workout, or a fun-filled adventure with friends or loved ones, a nutritious smoothie can help you stay focused and fully engaged.

All too often, we choose to fuel our bodies with processed foods that contain lots of calories and fat. Unfortunately, even fortified snack foods are missing important nutrients that help the body and mind to perform properly. If you're accustomed to using energy drinks, coffee, or sugary sodas to boost your energy, you know how quickly the body crashes after the initial power surge wears off. This happens because many energy supplements are missing fiber and fat—both of which slow digestion and prevent sugars and other nutrients from being absorbed too rapidly.

By replacing sugary beverages and other undesirable options with whole, natural fruits and vegetables, you provide yourself with nutrients that contribute to sustained energy, such as B vitamins and chlorophyll. As the modern diet often contains less fresh food than it should, these nutrients are often completely missing or consumed in smaller quantities than nature intended. Start consuming them in abundance, and you'll notice an almost instant feeling of vitality.

Superfoods are also excellent sources of energy, as they contain high levels of essential enzymes and other nutrients that work in concert with the foods we eat, promoting complete digestion and absorption of the goodness found in natural foods. Smoothies containing superfoods and other supplements taste nearly identical to those without them, so feel free to transform any of the smoothies in this book into a powerful energy drink. You'll find plenty of tips for using superfoods in this chapter, and the more often you enjoy these smoothies, the easier it will be for you to make modifications and create your own delicious concoctions.

Reduce caffeine consumption—Caffeine is a naturally occurring stimulant. While small amounts of caffeine are not harmful, this addictive substance can be detrimental to your health when consumed in large amounts. Reducing your caffeine intake can help reduce blood pressure, leading to improved heart health, and it can also improve your body's ability to absorb calcium, leading to stronger bones. To eliminate uncomfortable side effects such as headaches and irritability, cut back slowly. Over time, you'll notice that you are sleeping better and that your natural energy level improves.

Berry-Almond Body Builder

YIELDS 4 CUPS

▶ 98 CALORIES PER CUP

Almonds offer an abundance of nutrients for sustained energy, including vitamin B-6, potassium, selenium, and protein. They also contain plenty of monounsaturated fat, which helps your body absorb carbohydrates at an even pace while promoting cardiovascular health. Bananas and berries are brimming with the natural goodness your body needs to rise to whatever challenges come your way.

You can transform this smoothie by using any of your favorite fruits in place of the mixed berries. Peaches, apricots, nectarines, and mangos are all delicious with almonds.

1 CUP UNSWEETENED ALMOND MILK

1 BANANA, PEELED AND CUT INTO 1-INCH CHUNKS

2 CUPS FROZEN MIXED BERRIES

¼ CUP RAW OR BLANCHED ALMONDS

4 ICE CUBES

1. Combine the almond milk and banana in the blender and process until smooth.

2. Add the berries and almonds, pulsing and blending until well incorporated.

3. Add the ice cubes and blend until the desired consistency has been achieved.

4. Spoon or pour into a glass and enjoy.

Tropical Muscle Machine

YIELDS 4 CUPS

▶ 136 CALORIES PER CUP

Often referred to as the "king of fruits," mango is wonderfully nutritious with a delightfully buttery texture and a flavor that's difficult to beat. High in potassium, vitamin A, alpha and beta carotene, and other nutrients, this tropical fruit is a favorite all over the world. Bright red raspberries and goji berries increase this recipe's antioxidant content, while almond milk and protein powder provide satisfaction that lasts for hours.

1 CUP UNSWEETENED ALMOND MILK
1 BANANA, PEELED AND CUT INTO 1-INCH CHUNKS
1 CUP FRESH OR FROZEN MANGO CHUNKS
1 CUP FRESH OR FROZEN RASPBERRIES
¼ CUP DRIED GOJI BERRIES
1 SCOOP VANILLA-FLAVORED PROTEIN POWDER
¼ TEASPOON PURE VANILLA EXTRACT
8 ICE CUBES

1. Combine the almond milk and banana in the blender, processing until smooth.

2. Add the mango, raspberries, goji berries, protein powder, and vanilla, then blend and pulse until well incorporated.

3. Add the ice cubes and blend until the desired consistency has been achieved.

4. Spoon or pour into a glass and enjoy.

Purple Protein Pick-Me-Up

▶ 88 CALORIES PER CUP

All body tissues, including hair and nails, contain at least a little protein. Known as the building block of life, protein is a nutrient no one can do without. Plants contain an abundance of protein, and as science has proven, it's possible to consume an entirely plant-based diet without causing harm to the body. This vegan protein shake is perfectly delicious, and it's nutritious enough to power you through even the toughest workout.

When shopping for tofu, choose a brand that doesn't contain GMO soy, if possible. While discussions are ongoing as to whether GMO foods are harmful to human health, it's best to err on the side of caution.

1 CUP UNSWEETENED ALMOND MILK
4 OUNCES SILKEN TOFU
1 BANANA, PEELED AND CUT INTO 1-INCH CHUNKS
3 CUPS FRESH OR FROZEN BLACKBERRIES
STEVIA EXTRACT
8 ICE CUBES

1. Combine the almond milk, tofu, and banana in the blender, processing until smooth.

2. Add the blackberries, stevia to taste, and ice cubes, then blend and pulse until all ingredients have been thoroughly incorporated.

3. Spoon or pour into a glass and enjoy.

Peachy Banana Protein Power

YIELDS 4 CUPS

125 CALORIES PER CUP

Bee pollen isn't just a source of essential vitamins and minerals; it also contains an abundance of protein and more than five thousand enzymes. Perfect for pairing with peaches and vanilla-flavored protein powder, bee pollen and honey are at their best when sourced from apiaries near you, as they tend to be fresher and may even help to ward off seasonal allergies.

If fresh peaches or nectarines aren't in season, you can use frozen peach slices or 2 cups of your favorite fruit.

1 CUP UNSWEETENED ALMOND MILK

1 BANANA, PEELED AND CUT INTO 1-INCH CHUNKS

3 PEACHES OR NECTARINES, PITTED AND CUT INTO 1-INCH CHUNKS

1 SCOOP VANILLA-FLAVORED PROTEIN POWDER

1 TABLESPOON LOCAL BEE POLLEN

1 TABLESPOON LOCAL HONEY

¼ TEASPOON PURE VANILLA EXTRACT

8 ICE CUBES

1. Combine the almond milk and banana in the blender and process until smooth.

2. Add the peaches, protein powder, bee pollen, honey, and vanilla, then pulse and blend until all ingredients have been fully incorporated.

3. Add the ice cubes, continuing to pulse and blend until the desired texture has been achieved.

4. Spoon or pour into a glass and enjoy.

Berry-Vanilla Vitality

▶ 110 CALORIES PER CUP

Antioxidant-rich camu camu berry is perhaps best known for its link to eye health, but it's also the perfect superfood for retaining mental clarity. This smoothie also contains protein, carbohydrates, and a small amount of healthy fat to keep you feeling satisfied and focused on the task at hand.

This recipe works perfectly with any of your favorite berries, including frozen berry blends commonly found in supermarkets.

1 CUP UNSWEETENED ALMOND MILK

1 BANANA, PEELED AND CUT INTO 1-INCH CHUNKS

2 CUPS FRESH OR FROZEN RASPBERRIES

1 SCOOP VANILLA-FLAVORED PROTEIN POWDER

1 TABLESPOON POWDERED CAMU CAMU BERRY

¼ TEASPOON PURE VANILLA EXTRACT

8 ICE CUBES

1. Combine the almond milk and banana in the blender and process until smooth.

2. Add the raspberries, protein powder, powdered camu camu berry, and vanilla, then pulse and blend until all ingredients have been thoroughly combined.

3. Add the ice cubes and process until the desired consistency has been achieved.

4. Spoon or pour into a glass and enjoy.

Extra-Berry Energy

YIELDS 6 CUPS

▶ 65 CALORIES PER CUP

For more than two thousand years, Peruvians have been using maca root to provide them with the endurance and strength required for challenging physical activities. Powdered maca root is also linked to healthy libido, balanced mood, and overall vitality, making it a superfood with some truly enjoyable benefits.

You can substitute 4 cups of any of your favorite fruit for the berries to change this smoothie's flavor.

1 CUP UNSWEETENED ALMOND MILK
1 BANANA, PEELED AND CUT INTO 1-INCH CHUNKS
1 TEASPOON MACA ROOT POWDER
2 CUPS FRESH STRAWBERRIES
2 CUPS MIXED FROZEN BERRIES
8 ICE CUBES

1. Combine the almond milk, banana, and maca root powder in the blender, processing until smooth.

2. Add the strawberries and mixed berries, pulsing and blending until smooth.

3. Incorporate the ice, processing until the desired consistency has been achieved.

4. Spoon or pour into a glass and enjoy.

Green Gumption

▶ 86 CALORIES PER CUP

Not only is chlorella an excellent superfood for energy, with plenty of protein, vitamins, and minerals—plus more chlorophyll than any other known plant—but it's also a natural detoxifier.

Be sure to choose a brand that is raw and organic, and check that the packaging specifies that it has broken cell walls. Other types of chlorella are often less expensive but cannot be fully absorbed by the body.

1 CUP CHILLED GREEN TEA

1 BANANA, PEELED AND CUT INTO 1-INCH CHUNKS

1 CUP ORGANIC GREEN GRAPES

3 KIWI FRUIT, PEELED AND HALVED

1 CUP FRESH HONEYDEW MELON CHUNKS

3 TABLESPOONS CHLORELLA POWDER

1 CUP CHOPPED BABY SPINACH, LOOSELY PACKED

1 CUP CHOPPED ROMAINE LETTUCE, LOOSELY PACKED

8 ICE CUBES

1. Combine the tea and banana in the blender and process until smooth.

2. Add the grapes, kiwi, honeydew, and chlorella powder, then pulse and blend until well incorporated.

3. Add the spinach and romaine, processing until smooth, then add the ice cubes and blend until the desired consistency has been achieved.

4. Spoon or pour into a glass and enjoy.

Spirulina Power Punch

YIELDS 4 CUPS

▶ 76 CALORIES PER CUP

Spirulina consists of 65 percent protein—the highest percentage that any plant contains—and it also has eighteen amino acids, including the eight that are essential to human health. Not only does it provide energy that's easy for the body to absorb, but it also supplies tryptophan, which aids in building serotonin, a brain chemical that elevates mood and promotes restful sleep. An excellent superfood for anyone who is trying to cut back on caffeine, spirulina provides an almost instant burst of energy.

If you still need a little caffeine, replace the peach tea with green, white, or black tea. This will increase the amount of energy in the smoothie and give you an antioxidant boost as well.

1 CUP CHILLED PEACH-FLAVORED HERBAL TEA
1 BANANA, PEELED AND CUT INTO 1-INCH CHUNKS
3 NECTARINES, PITTED AND QUARTERED
3 APRICOTS, PITTED AND HALVED
1 TABLESPOON SPIRULINA POWDER
1 CUP CHOPPED BUTTER LETTUCE, LOOSELY PACKED
8 ICE CUBES

1. Combine the tea and banana in the blender, processing until smooth.

2. Add the nectarines, apricots, and spirulina powder, blending again until smooth.

3. Incorporate the butter lettuce and ice cubes, pulsing and blending until the desired consistency has been achieved.

4. Pour into a glass and enjoy.

Mango-Peach Supreme

YIELDS 4 CUPS

▶ 99 CALORIES PER CUP

Hemp seed is one of the best sources of plant protein available, with more protein per serving than seeds, nuts, and all other plants with the exception of spirulina. An excellent energy supplement that aids in healthy muscle growth and tissue repair, food-grade hemp seed doesn't come from the cannabis plant, though it's a close relative. With twenty amino acids including the eight essentials, it's also an excellent source of omega-3 and omega-6 fatty acids, antioxidants, vitamins, and minerals. One of the easiest ways to include it in your diet is to choose an organic hemp protein powder like the one this recipe calls for.

Note: If you are subject to drug testing during the course of employment, avoid hemp in any form as it can sometimes cause a false positive for marijuana. Simply choose a different type of protein powder and add a tablespoon of powdered flaxseed to this recipe.

1 CUP UNSWEETENED ALMOND MILK

1 BANANA, PEELED AND CUT INTO 1-INCH CHUNKS

1 CUP FRESH OR FROZEN MANGO CHUNKS

1 PEACH OR NECTARINE, PITTED AND QUARTERED

1 CUP FRESH OR FROZEN STRAWBERRIES

1 SCOOP ORGANIC HEMP PROTEIN POWDER

8 ICE CUBES

1. Combine the almond milk and banana in the blender and process until smooth.

2. Add the mango, peach or nectarine, strawberries, and protein powder, then pulse and blend until fully incorporated.

3. Add the ice cubes, pulsing and blending until the desired consistency has been reached.

4. Pour into a glass and enjoy.

Veggie Verve

YIELDS 5 CUPS

▶ 63 CALORIES PER CUP

Also known as kombu, kelp has a somewhat strong taste that might remind you of the salty scent of the ocean and is best used in smoothie recipes that contain savory ingredients. It's an excellent source of minerals and an outstanding source of iodine, which is essential for thyroid health. With vitamins and trace elements that help keep the body energized, kelp is a wonderful addition to the diet.

Adjust the amount of jalapeño as you please; if you like very hot, spicy flavors, try adding twice the amount this recipe calls for and continuing to increase the heat if desired.

1 CUP CHILLED GREEN TEA

1 MEDIUM ORGANIC CUCUMBER, PEEL ON, CUT INTO
    1-INCH SEGMENTS

2 MEDIUM ORGANIC CARROTS, PEELED, CUT INTO
    1-INCH SEGMENTS

2 LARGE ORGANIC VINE-RIPENED TOMATOES, QUARTERED

3 RIBS ORGANIC CELERY, LONG FIBROUS STRANDS REMOVED,
    CUT INTO 1-INCH SEGMENTS

1 ORGANIC GREEN, YELLOW, OR RED BELL PEPPER, SEEDED
    AND QUARTERED

1 TEASPOON KELP POWDER

1 TABLESPOON CHLORELLA POWDER

1 CUP CHOPPED ORGANIC BABY SPINACH, LOOSELY PACKED

¼ CUP FRESH CILANTRO LEAVES, LOOSELY PACKED
½ JALAPEÑO PEPPER, SEEDED AND CUT INTO 1-INCH SEGMENTS
JUICE FROM 1 LIME
8 ICE CUBES

1. Combine the tea, cucumber, carrots, tomatoes, celery, bell pepper, kelp powder, and chlorella in the blender, processing until smooth.

2. Add the spinach, cilantro, jalapeño, lime juice, and ice cubes, and process again until all ingredients have been fully incorporated. Leave the blender closed for about 30 seconds after processing to allow any airborne jalapeño juice to settle, as it can irritate your eyes and nasal passages.

3. Pour into a glass and enjoy.

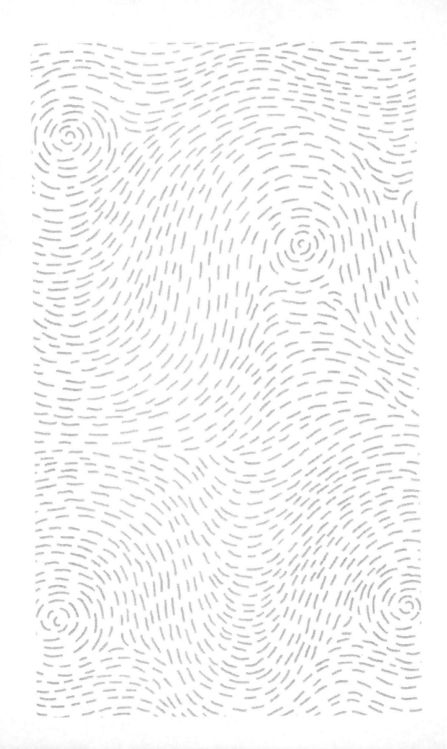

CHAPTER TEN

Detox and Cleanse

Toxins are all around us. Not only are they present in many of the foods we eat and in much of the water we drink, but they are also in the air we breathe, the cleaning products we use in our homes and businesses, the gasoline we put in our cars, and even the hygiene products we apply to our bodies each day.

It's important to avoid exposure to as many of these toxins as possible. You can greatly reduce your own toxin levels by eating organic foods; avoiding fish known to contain high levels of heavy metal including mercury; avoiding fatty meats from feedlot animals and those raised in confinement on factory farms and fed toxic diets; and using nontoxic cleaning and hygiene products. It's also best to drink filtered water rather than water straight from the tap or bottled water from plastic containers that are manufactured with poisonous chemical additives like BPA.

Even when we do take all of these steps and do our best to avoid substances like food additives, nicotine, and excessive alcohol, we're still exposed to environmental toxins. One of the best ways to eliminate these toxins and keep them from building up in our bodies is to drink smoothies that contain ingredients known for their ability to cleanse and detoxify the body.

Each of the recipes in this chapter contains ingredients known for their ability to help draw toxins from the body. While it's vital that you eat as many organic fruits and vegetables as possible each day, it's even more important that you choose organic options when cleansing your body.

Enjoy a weekend detox—*Many people turn to spas and wellness resorts for detoxification, and for good reasons: these venues provide healthful cleansing and detox menus while offering an abundance of desirable services including massages, pedicures, exercise classes, meditation, and plenty of quiet time. If you're planning to do a three-day detox, why not treat yourself to some pampering? Schedule a massage and a pedicure, take long baths, catch up on your reading, and give yourself time to meditate, write in a journal, or just relax and unwind. If you have children, consider asking grandparents or other relatives to take them for the weekend even if all you plan to do is stay home. Quiet time is vital to healthy detox, particularly if you live a fast-paced lifestyle.*

Green Berry Detox Blast

YIELDS 5 CUPS

▶ 41 CALORIES PER CUP

Organic berries contain plenty of water, which aids in flushing toxins from the body. They're filled with nutrients, including powerful antioxidants that help cells repair the damage that toxins can do. In addition, they're very easy to digest, freeing up your liver and kidneys for the important task of eliminating toxic substances from your body.

This recipe works well with either fresh or frozen organic berries, so you can make it even when fresh local berries are out of season.

1 CUP CHILLED FILTERED WATER
1 CUP ORGANIC STRAWBERRIES
1 CUP ORGANIC BLUEBERRIES
1 CUP ORGANIC BLACKBERRIES
2 CUPS ORGANIC BABY SPINACH, CHOPPED AND
    LOOSELY PACKED
8 ICE CUBES MADE WITH FILTERED WATER

1. Combine the water, strawberries, blueberries, and blackberries in the blender, processing until smooth.

2. Add the spinach and ice cubes, blending and pulsing until all ingredients have been well incorporated.

3. Pour into a glass and enjoy.

Carrot Cleanse

YIELDS 3 CUPS

▶ 111 CALORIES PER CUP

Citrus fruits are powerful detoxification agents. Not only are they high in vital nutrients that support the body and rebuild tissues during the cleansing process, but they also contain an abundance of fiber that helps to sweep your intestines clean, moving trapped toxins out of the digestive tract. Carrots contain even more fiber and nutrients, plus they give this smoothie a pleasant texture while mellowing the citrus flavors.

1 CUP CHILLED FILTERED WATER
2 ORGANIC CARROTS, PEELED AND CUT INTO 1-INCH SEGMENTS
1 ORGANIC GRAPEFRUIT, PEELED, SEEDED, AND SECTIONED
2 ORGANIC VALENCIA ORANGES, PEELED, SEEDED,
    AND SECTIONED
¼ ORGANIC LEMON, PEELED AND SEEDED
8 ICE CUBES MADE WITH FILTERED WATER
ORGANIC STEVIA EXTRACT (OPTIONAL)

1. Combine the water and carrots in the blender and process until smooth.

2. Add the grapefruit, oranges, and lemon, blending until smooth.

3. Add the ice cubes, blending and pulsing until all ingredients have been well incorporated and the desired consistency has been achieved.

4. If the taste of this smoothie is too tart, add a few drops of organic stevia extract to taste.

5. Pour into a glass and enjoy.

Ginger Detox Delight

YIELDS 3 CUPS

▶ 79 CALORIES PER CUP

Fresh ginger stimulates the digestive system so that toxins are elimi-
nated faster, and it gives smoothies a very appealing taste. If you like
the flavor of fresh ginger in your smoothies, be sure to try adding it to
other recipes. It's excellent with fruits such as apples, pears, pineapple,
and citrus.

1 CUP CHILLED FILTERED WATER
1 ORGANIC PEAR, CORED AND CUT INTO 1-INCH CHUNKS
2 ORGANIC GRANNY SMITH APPLES, CORED AND CUT INTO
    1-INCH CHUNKS
½-INCH PIECE OF ORGANIC GINGER ROOT, PEELED AND
    CHOPPED OR THINLY SLICED
1 CUP CHOPPED ORGANIC ROMAINE LETTUCE, LOOSELY PACKED
8 ICE CUBES MADE WITH FILTERED WATER

1. Combine the water and pear in the blender, processing until smooth.

2. Add the apples and ginger, pulsing and blending until smooth.

3. Add the romaine and ice cubes, continuing to pulse and blend until all ingredients have been well incorporated and the desired consistency has been achieved.

4. Pour into a glass and enjoy.

Spicy Tomato-Cucumber Cleanse

YIELDS 5 CUPS

▶ 31 CALORIES PER CUP

Cayenne pepper offers a powerful detoxification effect: it serves as a diuretic, aids in eliminating built-up fecal matter, removes undesirable bacteria from the gut, and even helps to detoxify the cardiovascular system by repairing damaged blood cells and aiding in the removal of plaque that has accumulated in the arteries.

If you're sensitive to hot spices, use just a pinch of cayenne pepper and slowly increase the amount as needed.

1 CUP CHILLED FILTERED WATER

1 LARGE ORGANIC CUCUMBER, PEEL ON, CUT INTO
    1-INCH SEGMENTS

3 LARGE ORGANIC VINE-RIPENED TOMATOES, QUARTERED

3 STALKS ORGANIC CELERY, LONG FIBERS REMOVED,
    CUT INTO 1-INCH SEGMENTS

½ TEASPOON CAYENNE PEPPER

JUICE FROM 1 ORGANIC LIME

8 ICE CUBES MADE WITH FILTERED WATER

1. Combine the water and cucumber in the blender, processing until smooth.

2. Add the tomatoes, celery, cayenne pepper, and lime juice, then blend and pulse until well incorporated.

3. Add the ice cubes, blending and pulsing until the desired consistency has been achieved.

4. Pour into a glass and enjoy.

Mellow Mango

YIELDS 3 CUPS

▶ 80 CALORIES PER CUP

Green tea contains high levels of antioxidants including catechins, which contribute to healthy liver function. In addition, it acts as a mild diuretic, helping to draw contaminants out of the body by increasing urine production. Be sure to use filtered water to make the tea for this smoothie, and consider permanently replacing potentially toxic tap and bottled water with filtered.

1 CUP CHILLED GREEN TEA MADE WITH FILTERED WATER
1 ORGANIC BANANA, PEELED AND CUT INTO 1-INCH CHUNKS
1 CUP ORGANIC MANGO CHUNKS
1 ORGANIC PEACH, PITTED AND HALVED
8 ICE CUBES MADE WITH FILTERED WATER

1. Combine the tea and banana in the blender and process until smooth.

2. Add the mango, peach, and ice cubes, blending and pulsing until the desired consistency has been achieved.

3. Pour into a glass and enjoy.

Cleansing Cucumber

YIELDS 4 CUPS

▶ 47 CALORIES PER CUP

Cucumbers contain very few calories, yet they are brimming with nutrients that aid in healthy detoxification. Rich in potassium, phosphorus, and sodium, they are naturally hydrating; however, they do act as a mild diuretic, promoting the rapid elimination of contaminants. As cucumbers have a very mild taste, they are ideal for adding to any of your favorite smoothie recipes.

This recipe is delicious with any type of fruit, so if you can't find organic honeydew melon, replace it with an organic fruit that's easier to find in your area.

1 CUP CHILLED FILTERED WATER
2 ORGANIC CUCUMBERS, PEELS ON, CUT INTO 1-INCH SEGMENTS
2 CUPS ORGANIC HONEYDEW MELON CHUNKS
1 CUP CHOPPED ORGANIC ROMAINE LETTUCE, LOOSELY PACKED
8 ICE CUBES MADE WITH FILTERED WATER

1. Combine the water and cucumbers in the blender, processing until smooth.

2. Add the honeydew and romaine, blending and pulsing until well incorporated.

3. Add the ice cubes and continue to blend until the desired consistency has been achieved.

4. Pour into a glass and enjoy.

Green Banana Detox

▶ 72 CALORIES PER CUP

Cup for cup, broccoli sprouts contain even more powerful antioxidants than full-grown broccoli does. These antioxidants work to stimulate the naturally occurring detoxification enzymes found in the body's digestive tract.

If you can't find broccoli sprouts in your local health food store, you can easily grow them from seed in a sunny window. Using a sprout-growing kit is one of the best ways to ensure that you'll never run out of fresh, wholesome greens for your smoothies.

This recipe can be easily customized to your personal taste; simply replace the berry blend with an equal amount of the fresh or frozen organic fruit of your choice.

1 CUP CHILLED GREEN TEA MADE WITH FILTERED WATER
1 ORGANIC BANANA, PEELED AND CUT INTO 1-INCH CHUNKS
3 CUPS ORGANIC FROZEN MIXED BERRIES
1 CUP ORGANIC BROCCOLI SPROUTS, LOOSELY PACKED

1. Combine the tea and banana in the blender and process until smooth.

2. Add the berries and broccoli sprouts, then pulse and blend until the desired consistency has been achieved.

3. Pour into a glass and enjoy.

Melon Cleanse

YIELDS 5 CUPS

▶ 25 CALORIES PER CUP

Watermelon is definitely delicious, and it's also a powerful detoxifying agent with the ability to help the liver process ammonia, which is a naturally occurring waste product that builds up as amino acids are metabolized. This juicy red fruit also contains high levels of lycopene, vitamin C, vitamin A, and fiber, making it an excellent addition to almost any smoothie.

This recipe is also fantastic with organic cantaloupe or honeydew melon, both of which contain some of the same detoxifying compounds that watermelon does.

1 CUP CHILLED FILTERED WATER
3 CUPS ORGANIC WATERMELON CHUNKS, WITH
    OR WITHOUT SEEDS
¼ LEMON, PEELED AND SEEDED
8 ICE CUBES MADE WITH FILTERED WATER

1. Combine the water, watermelon, and lemon in the blender, processing until smooth.

2. Add the ice cubes, blending and pulsing until well incorporated.

3. Pour into a glass and enjoy.

Detox Dream

YIELDS 5 CUPS

▶ 51 CALORIES PER CUP

Combine detoxifying fruits and vegetables to make smoothies that pull double duty. This blend makes the most of nutritious greens, citrus, watermelon, and cucumber, pleasing your palate while helping to clear your system of built-up waste.

If you dislike grapefruit or avoid it because of potential drug interactions, you can replace it with two organic Valencia oranges or four organic tangerines.

1 CUP CHILLED GREEN TEA MADE WITH FILTERED WATER
1 ORGANIC CUCUMBER, PEEL ON, CUT INTO 1-INCH SEGMENTS
1 ORGANIC GRAPEFRUIT, PEELED, SEEDED, AND SECTIONED
2 CUPS ORGANIC WATERMELON CHUNKS, WITH
    OR WITHOUT SEEDS
1 CUP CHOPPED ORGANIC BABY SPINACH, LOOSELY PACKED
8 ICE CUBES MADE WITH FILTERED WATER

1. Combine the tea and cucumber in the blender and process until smooth.

2. Add the grapefruit and watermelon, blending again until well incorporated, then add the spinach and blend once more.

3. Add the ice cubes, pulsing and blending until the desired consistency has been achieved.

4. Pour into a glass and enjoy.

Cherry Champion

YIELDS 4 CUPS

▶ 108 CALORIES PER CUP

Nutritious oils containing omega-3 fatty acids are ideal for consumption during a cleanse, as they help to keep intestinal walls lubricated, and toxins are absorbed by the oils for easy expulsion from the body. Avocado oil, flaxseed oil, olive oil, and hemp oil are all good choices.

This recipe works well with either fresh or frozen sweet cherries. If you don't have cherries, simply use an equal amount of any organic fruit you have on hand.

1 CUP CHILLED FILTERED WATER
1 TABLESPOON ORGANIC FLAXSEED OIL
1 ORGANIC BANANA, PEELED AND CUT INTO 1-INCH CHUNKS
2 CUPS ORGANIC SWEET CHERRIES, PITTED AND STEMMED
JUICE FROM 1 ORGANIC LEMON
8 ICE CUBES MADE WITH FILTERED WATER

1. Combine the water, flaxseed oil, and banana in the blender, processing until smooth.

2. Add the cherries and lemon juice, pulsing and blending until well incorporated.

3. Add the ice cubes and continue to pulse and blend until the desired consistency has been achieved.

4. Pour into a glass and enjoy.

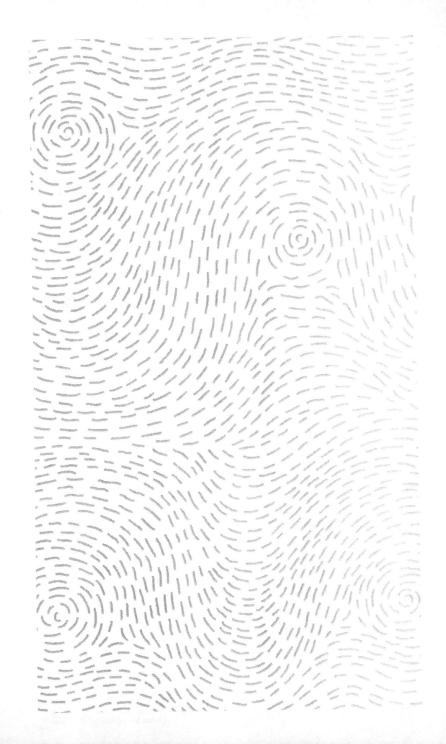

CHAPTER ELEVEN

Dessert Smoothies

As the popular saying goes, "Life is short, so eat dessert first." Unfortunately, an overabundance of unhealthy desserts containing high-fructose corn syrup, lots of fat, and far too many empty calories do nothing more than contribute to waistline expansion. Often addictive and difficult to consume in moderation, many popular desserts are best left alone.

Even so, it's possible to enjoy dessert while you lose weight, particularly when you choose healthy dessert smoothies that offer delightful flavors and an abundance of nutrients that don't normally make their way into traditional desserts. With ingredients such as chocolate, peanut butter, and even holiday eggnog, the smoothies in this chapter are definitely higher in calories and fat than the rest of the recipes this book contains; however, they're much healthier than other dessert options and can be safely enjoyed by anyone—even those who have extra pounds to shed.

Whether you're counting calories or simply longing for an alternative to a dessert you'd rather not consume due to health concerns, these quick, simple smoothies have been designed with you in mind. Ready in just a few minutes and brimming with healthy alternatives to traditional ingredients such as butter, cream, and refined sugar, these smoothies taste fantastic and are certain to be appreciated, even by those who have never tried smoothies. Present them in beautiful glasses and garnish them artfully for special occasions, or put them in simple mugs for everyday enjoyment. They're marvelously enjoyable either way.

Try variations on old favorites—*The dessert smoothie recipes in this chapter are delicious and will help you beat cravings for unhealthy options. Even so, you may find yourself craving a specific dessert you love. If you're not willing to compromise your healthy eating plan by consuming the dessert that has you under its spell, try creating a smoothie that incorporates its flavors—it just may do the trick. Don't beat yourself up if you end up giving in, particularly on a special occasion. A healthy, sustainable diet is one that allows for the occasional treat, whether that's a dessert smoothie or a piece of your favorite aunt's famous carrot cake.*

Bananas Foster

▶ 122 CALORIES PER CUP

Traditional bananas foster is delicious, but it's loaded with butter, sugary liqueur, and an abundance of highly processed sugar. This smoothie is brimming with tasty bananas and contains natural vanilla as well as a touch of evaporated cane juice and cinnamon to impart warm sweetness.

1 CUP CHAI SPICE TEA
4 BANANAS, PEELED AND CUT INTO 1-INCH CHUNKS
1 TEASPOON CINNAMON
¼ CUP ORGANIC EVAPORATED SUGAR CANE JUICE
   (OFTEN MARKETED AS SUGAR IN THE RAW)
½ TEASPOON PURE VANILLA EXTRACT
8 ICE CUBES

1. Combine the tea and bananas in the blender, processing until smooth. Add a little more tea or water if the blades start to stick.

2. Add the cinnamon, sugar cane juice, and vanilla, blending again until well incorporated.

3. Add the ice cubes, pulsing and blending until the desired consistency has been achieved.

4. Spoon or pour into four glasses and serve.

Holiday Eggnog

▶ 227 CALORIES PER CUP

Nothing says "holiday" quite like eggnog. This smoothie is perfect for serving to guests as a light but sweet dessert after a heavy meal and is very easy to make in advance. Try freezing it in small dishes for a treat that's a bit healthier than some other popular holiday dessert options.

2 CUPS EGGNOG OR DAIRY-FREE EGGNOG
2 BANANAS, PEELED AND CUT INTO 1-INCH CHUNKS
1 TEASPOON PURE VANILLA EXTRACT
8 ICE CUBES
GROUND OR FRESHLY GRATED NUTMEG FOR GARNISH

1. Combine the eggnog and bananas in the blender, processing until smooth.

2. Add the vanilla and ice cubes, pulsing and blending until fully incorporated.

3. Pour into four glasses, garnish with a sprinkle of nutmeg, and serve.

Tangerine Temptation

▶ 190 CALORIES PER CUP

Tangerines have a taste that's often much sweeter than that of other citrus fruits, making them the perfect choice for use in dessert smoothies. This recipe contains healthy protein and no processed sugar, making it a great choice for inclusion in a weight loss plan.

For an even frostier treat, freeze the banana chunks and tangerine sections in advance.

1 CUP UNSWEETENED ALMOND MILK

2 BANANAS, PEELED AND CUT INTO 1-INCH CHUNKS

10 TANGERINES OR CLEMENTINES, PEELED, SEEDED, AND SECTIONED

1 TEASPOON PURE VANILLA EXTRACT

5 DROPS STEVIA EXTRACT

8 ICE CUBES

1. Combine the almond milk and bananas in the blender, processing until smooth.

2. Add the tangerines, then blend and pulse until fully incorporated.

3. Add the vanilla, stevia, and ice cubes, blending and pulsing until the desired consistency has been reached.

4. Pour into four glasses and serve immediately.

Chocolate-Peppermint Delight

YIELDS 4 CUPS

▶ 72 CALORIES PER CUP

Chocolate and peppermint are delicious any time of year, but many treats that feature this delightful flavor combination are woefully high in calories, contain highly processed ingredients, and do nothing to benefit health. This light yet flavorful recipe gets its minty fresh taste from pure peppermint essential oil, which offers numerous health benefits and aids in promoting healthy digestion.

2 CUPS CHOCOLATE-FLAVORED ALMOND MILK, DIVIDED

4 TABLESPOONS PURE UNSWEETENED COCOA POWDER

¼ TEASPOON PURE VANILLA EXTRACT

8 DROPS STEVIA EXTRACT

2 DROPS FOOD-GRADE PEPPERMINT ESSENTIAL OIL

12 ICE CUBES

FRESH MINT LEAVES FOR GARNISH (OPTIONAL)

1. Combine ¼ cup of the chocolate almond milk with the cocoa powder in the blender and process for 30 seconds. Add another ¼ cup of chocolate almond milk, and repeat, pulsing and blending until the cocoa powder is well incorporated.

2. Add the remaining 1½ cups of chocolate almond milk, vanilla, stevia, and peppermint essential oil, along with the ice cubes. Pulse and blend until the ice cubes have been fully incorporated.

3. Spoon or pour into four glasses and serve. Garnish with fresh mint leaves if you like.

Luscious Lemon

YIELDS 4 CUPS

▶ 68 CALORIES PER CUP

Lemons have a light, refreshing flavor that cleanses the palate while providing just a little satisfying sweetness. Unlike many classic lemon desserts, which are often high in sugar and fat, this smoothie has very few calories and comes with some health benefits, thanks to vitamin C and other nutrients that give lemons their zippy flavor.

If you enjoy fruity lemon treats, try adding a cup of frozen strawberries, cherries, or raspberries to the blender just before incorporating the ice cubes.

1 CUP CHILLED WATER
2 BANANAS, PEELED AND CUT INTO 1-INCH CHUNKS
3 LEMONS, PEELED, SEEDED, AND SECTIONED
½ TEASPOON PURE VANILLA EXTRACT
16 TO 20 DROPS STEVIA EXTRACT
20 ICE CUBES

1. Combine the water and bananas in the blender and process until smooth.

2. Add the lemons, vanilla, stevia, and ice cubes, pulsing and blending until smooth. Adjust the amount of stevia to suit your taste.

3. Pour or spoon into four glasses and serve.

Banana Split

▶ 138 CALORIES PER CUP

An indulgent banana split gets most of its flavor from the fruit toppings, not from the fat-filled ice cream it contains. This healthy banana split smoothie tastes fantastic, whether you decide to serve it with or without a little vanilla ice cream. Top with a small amount of whipped topping, a splash of chocolate syrup, and a maraschino cherry for an even richer treat.

1 CUP UNSWEETENED ALMOND MILK
2 BANANAS, PEELED AND CUT INTO 1-INCH CHUNKS
½ CUP FROZEN STRAWBERRIES
1 CUP FRESH OR FROZEN PINEAPPLE CHUNKS
3 TABLESPOONS LOCAL HONEY
½ TEASPOON PURE VANILLA EXTRACT
12 ICE CUBES

1. Combine the almond milk and bananas in the blender, processing until smooth.

2. Add the strawberries and pineapple, pulsing and blending until fully incorporated.

3. Add the honey, vanilla, and ice cubes, continuing to pulse and blend until the desired consistency has been achieved.

4. Pour into four glasses and enjoy.

Sweet Vanilla Bean

YIELDS 4 CUPS

▶ 203 CALORIES PER CUP

Vanilla, oranges, and bananas come together perfectly in this delicious dessert smoothie, which is truly decadent and perfect for serving to guests. If you don't do dairy or dislike the idea of using full-fat ice cream, simply replace the ice cream with vanilla-flavored yogurt or nondairy yogurt, or substitute it with vanilla-flavored nondairy ice cream.

1 CUP MILK OR NONDAIRY MILK
2 CUPS PREMIUM VANILLA BEAN ICE CREAM
1 BANANA, PEELED AND CUT INTO 1-INCH CHUNKS
½ CUP FRESHLY SQUEEZED ORANGE JUICE
½ TEASPOON PURE VANILLA EXTRACT

1. Combine the milk, ice cream, and banana in the blender, processing until incorporated.

2. Add the orange juice and vanilla, blending and pulsing just until all ingredients have been combined.

3. Pour into four glasses and serve immediately.

Purple Cow

▶ 204 CALORIES PER CUP

A classic purple cow is basically an ice cream float made with grape soda—tasty, but not terribly healthy. This delicious smoothie contains plenty of fruit, vanilla, and classic ice cream minus the added sugar, artificial flavors, and artificial colors found in most commercially produced grape drinks.

If you don't do dairy or don't want to use full-fat ice cream, replace the ice cream with vanilla-flavored yogurt or nondairy yogurt, frozen yogurt, or dairy-free ice cream. The flavor will be just as enjoyable, and you'll be able to stick to your healthy diet.

½ CUP UNSWEETENED ALMOND OR DAIRY MILK
½ CUP GRAPE JUICE WITH NO SUGAR ADDED
2 CUPS PREMIUM VANILLA BEAN ICE CREAM
1 CUP FROZEN PURPLE GRAPES
1 CUP FROZEN BLACKBERRIES
½ TEASPOON PURE VANILLA EXTRACT

1. Combine the almond milk, grape juice, and ice cream in the blender, processing until smooth.

2. Add the grapes, blackberries, and vanilla, blending and pulsing until all ingredients have been incorporated.

3. Pour into four glasses and serve immediately.

Chocolate-Raspberry Mousse

YIELDS 4 CUPS

▶ 102 CALORIES PER CUP

Many decadent desserts feature the delicious flavor combination of raspberries and chocolate, but most of them have high levels of fat, cholesterol, and added sugar. Both raspberries and chocolate contain healthy antioxidants, vitamins, and fiber, making them great additions to a healthy diet.

2 CUPS CHOCOLATE-FLAVORED ALMOND MILK, DIVIDED

4 TABLESPOONS UNSWEETENED COCOA POWDER

2 CUPS FROZEN RASPBERRIES

½ TEASPOON PURE VANILLA EXTRACT

8 DROPS STEVIA EXTRACT

1. Combine ¼ cup of the chocolate almond milk and the unsweetened cocoa powder in the blender, processing for 30 seconds. Blend in an additional ¼ cup of chocolate almond milk, processing for another 30 seconds or so.

2. Add the remaining 1½ cups of chocolate almond milk, along with the raspberries, vanilla, and stevia, blending until all ingredients have been fully incorporated.

3. Pour into four glasses and serve immediately, or re-freeze the smoothie for a few hours, then run it through the blender for about 30 seconds for a frosty treat.

Peanut Butter Pie

YIELDS 4 CUPS

▶ 182 CALORIES PER CUP

Peanut butter pie is a tasty treat, but this heavy dessert is often laden with hundreds of empty calories from sugar and fat. This delicious but healthful smoothie contains chocolate and peanut butter to provide you with the flavors you're craving, and it's tasty enough to serve to your guests.

2 BANANAS, PEELED AND CUT INTO 1-INCH CHUNKS
4 TABLESPOONS UNSWEETENED COCOA POWDER
2 CUPS CHOCOLATE-FLAVORED ALMOND MILK
4 TABLESPOONS NATURAL PEANUT BUTTER
½ TEASPOON PURE VANILLA EXTRACT
8 DROPS STEVIA EXTRACT
8 ICE CUBES

1. Toss the banana chunks and cocoa powder together and put them into the blender with the chocolate almond milk. Process until smooth.

2. Add the peanut butter, vanilla, stevia, and ice cubes, blending and pulsing until all ingredients have been incorporated.

3. Pour into four glasses and serve immediately.

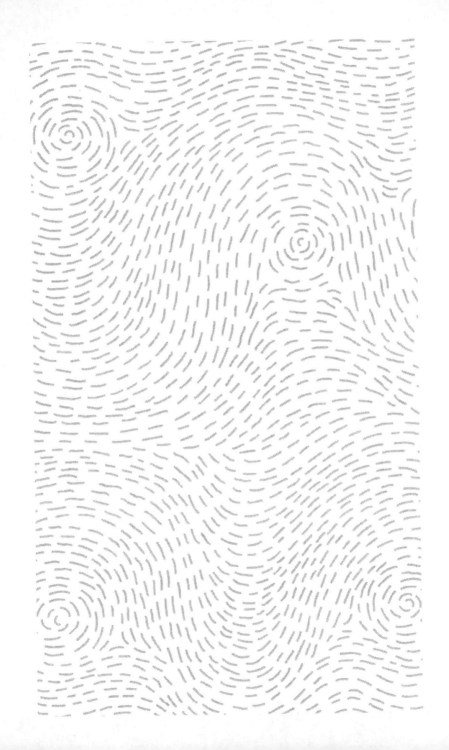

The Dirty Dozen and The Clean Fifteen

In an effort to increase food production and keep produce prices down, many farmers use conventional methods that include the application of chemical fertilizers and pesticides, despite the fact that many of these substances have been linked to cancer, birth defects, and other devastating health problems. According to the Environmental Working Group, an organization comprising researchers, policymakers, and scientists, you can reduce the amount of toxins in your daily diet by as much as 80 percent by consuming certain types of organic produce.

Using data from the United States Department of Agriculture (USDA) studies that focused on measuring the amount of toxic residue remaining on produce *after* it had been washed, the Environmental Working Group compiled two lists: The Dirty Dozen and The Clean Fifteen. These lists are intended to help consumers make purchasing decisions to prevent excessive exposure to toxic residues.

When conventionally grown, the fruits and vegetables comprising The Dirty Dozen list tested positive for as many as sixty-seven different chemicals and should be consumed only when organically grown. Those on The Clean Fifteen list bore little if any trace of chemical residue and are considered to be safe even when grown conventionally.

THE DIRTY DOZEN

Unfortunately, the dirty dozen list contains many of the best fruits and vegetables for health. Many of these are also popular smoothie ingredients.

- **Celery**—Celery grows in clumps, with the plants' bases forming cuplike reservoirs where moisture accumulates. Toxic residues also accumulate there, and celery is often completely coated in pesticide and herbicide with the heaviest concentrations being toward the bottom of the plant.
- **Peaches**—Peaches are very attractive to pests and are easily damaged, so farmers often feel the need to spray them heavily to prevent infestation. If you choose conventionally grown peaches, wash them well and peel them before use.
- **Strawberries**—Strawberries grow close to the ground and are targets for all sorts of pests. They also have bumpy exteriors with tiny hollows that allow residue to accumulate. As they won't hold up to heavy scrubbing and cannot be effectively peeled, it's best to choose organic ones or select a different fruit if an organic option is not available.
- **Apples**—Apples have concave areas at their stems and bud ends where toxic residue accumulates. Fortunately, they are easy to peel and core, so even if organic apples aren't an option, you can enjoy the inner portion of the fruit without worry. Keep in mind that there are many important nutrients in and just beneath an apple's skin; select organic whenever you can to get as many benefits as possible from this wonderful fruit.
- **Domestic Blueberries**—Like strawberries, blueberries are delicate and at risk of infestation. To keep prices down and increase yield, conventional growers utilize pesticides, which are very difficult to eliminate without destroying the berries. Organic blueberries are usually easy to find, particularly in the frozen food aisle.

- **Nectarines**—Nectarines attract pests and are easily damaged, so farmers often spray them heavily to prevent damage and potentially devastating crop losses. If you love nectarines and can't find organic ones, be sure to wash and peel them before consumption.
- **Peppers**—Both sweet and hot peppers are favorites with garden pests, so they're often liberally sprayed with a toxic cocktail of pesticides designed to prevent damage. Choose organic whenever possible.
- **Kale, Spinach, and Collard Greens**—Green vegetables like these are easy to grow organically, but many farmers elect to produce them conventionally. It's nearly impossible to rinse all the toxins off these essential foods, so be sure to choose organic at all times.
- **Cherries**—Sweet, delicate, and highly prized, cherries are easily damaged when bugs invade. The availability of fresh organic sweet cherries varies from one place to the next; if you cannot find them locally, you may need to select frozen organic sweet cherries.
- **Potatoes**—Potato bugs and other pests can rapidly devastate potato crops, so large-scale farmers often keep prices down by dousing their plants with pesticide that leach into the soil and into the potatoes. While you probably won't be adding potatoes to your smoothies, it's important to eat clean, healthy food at all times.
- **Grapes**—No matter what color they are, conventionally grown grapes—particularly those grown overseas—are covered in toxic pesticide. Organic producers are starting to offer more grape varieties, and these, along with organic grape juices and wines, are becoming easier to find in many places. If you cannot get organic grapes, choose a different fruit for your smoothies and snacks.

- **Lettuce**—Organic lettuce is now easy to find in most places, so whether you're enjoying a green smoothie or a salad, be sure to select an organic option rather than a conventional pesticide-laced one.

THE CLEAN FIFTEEN

Though this group of fruits and vegetables is considered safe to eat when grown conventionally, it's important to recognize that conventional agriculture practices are often not as sustainable as organic agricultural practices are. Choose organic foods whenever you can—you'll be promoting planetary health while doing your body a favor.

- **Onions**—Onions are not at all attractive to pests, so even those which are conventionally grown don't contain high levels of toxic residue. If you like green onions, look for an organic option so you can enjoy the tops as well as the bulbs.
- **Avocados**—With their thick skins, which are removed before consumption, avocados are a safe bet, whether grown conventionally or organically. Be sure to wash your avocados before cutting into them.
- **Pineapples**—Thick-skinned pineapples are another safe choice, even when conventionally grown.
- **Sweet Corn**—Even though you won't likely toss sweet corn into a smoothie, this vegetable is a delicious summertime treat that most people enjoy. Thanks to its husks, the kernels inside are not normally tainted with residual pesticide.
- **Mangos**—Like many other thick-skinned fruits and vegetables, mangos are fine to consume even if they have been conventionally grown. Be sure to remove all traces of skin before tossing fresh mango chunks into your smoothies.

- **Sweet Peas**—Thanks to their protective pods, sweet peas are a safe bet even when conventionally grown. They can be a fun addition to green smoothies, particularly when purchased fresh from the farmers' market.

- **Asparagus**—Pests do not care for asparagus, so it's not heavily doused with chemicals. While it's important to wash it before consumption, it's safe even if it's not organic.

- **Cabbage**—Only the outermost leaves of fresh cabbage are covered in pesticide; the inner leaves have been protected and are safe to consume. Avoid pre-shredded cabbage products though; these are less nutritious and more likely to be contaminated than whole cabbages are.

- **Kiwi Fruit**—As kiwi must be peeled before use, it's a good choice whether organically or conventionally grown. Wash it well before cutting or peeling to ensure no residue makes its way into the fruit's flesh.

- **Eggplant**—This member of the nightshade family is not terribly attractive to insects, so farmers often use very little pesticide. While raw eggplant is not suitable for addition to smoothies, cooked eggplant makes a great addition to a healthy diet.

- **Watermelon**—Watermelon's thick rind protects the fruit inside from pests, and even when pesticide has been heavily applied, it remains on the outside of the melon. Keep in mind that heirloom watermelon is often much tastier than its modern counterparts, and these old-fashioned melons are usually produced by organic farmers. Give them a try if you get an opportunity.

- **Cantaloupe**—Though cantaloupe has a thinner skin than watermelon does, its rinds protect the fruit inside from contamination. Due to the cantaloupe's texture, residue including potentially deadly bacteria accumulates easily. Be sure to scrub cantaloupes well under running water before cutting them open to avoid exposure to harmful toxins.

- **Grapefruit**—Grapefruit has a very thick skin that protects the flesh inside from being contaminated. Be sure to wash these fruits before peeling or cutting into them.
- **Sweet Potatoes**—Sweet potato vines are of little interest to insects, so farmers use fewer chemicals on them. Whether using them in smoothies or enjoying them for dinner, be sure to wash sweet potatoes and yams before using them.
- **Sweet Onions**—Like their pungent relatives, sweet onions are safe to enjoy whether conventionally or organically grown. Give them a try in savory smoothies—you may be pleasantly surprised.

It's important to remember that USDA testers measured toxin levels only after a thorough washing—and organic produce can still have traces of fertilizer, microbes, and other harmful substances on its skin, making proper decontamination a must. To reduce the potential that you'll ingest a harmful substance, be sure that you wash produce properly before eating it or putting it into your smoothies.

GROW YOUR OWN

In the days before commercial agriculture was prominent, almost everyone grew a few vegetables. Whether you've got room for a large garden or just a little space on a patio, you can easily grow some fresh produce of your own, eliminating many worries about pesticide and herbicide levels. Gardening is a great way to spend time outdoors, and it's also an excellent way to cut costs. Many of these vegetables and fruits are on the dirty dozen list but are very easy to grow, require little space, and provide even more nutrition if whipped up into smoothies immediately after harvest. Some to try include the following:

- **Greens**—All types of greens grow fairly quickly and require only a little care including regular watering. Lettuce, spinach, chard, and kale are all good options; grow them in stages by planting a small amount of seed each week for about a month. Harvest the plants when ready by cutting them, and in some cases, they'll keep on producing new leaves so you can enjoy a steady supply of fresh, organic greens with only a small investment of time and money.

- **Berries**—Strawberries are simple to grow in pots, hanging containers, and garden patches, and once established, blackberries, blueberries, and raspberries require little maintenance other than a bit of trimming and of course, some rewarding berry picking sessions. Protect your berries from birds by covering the plants with netting, and help keep bugs away by planting marigolds nearby.

- **Peppers**—Whether you like sweet peppers or hot varieties, you'll find that peppers are very easy to grow if you live in an area with warm summers. Start your plants indoors and transplant them after the last frost, either into pots, raised beds, a straw bale garden, or directly into the ground. Plant them close enough to one another so that their leaves will touch when mature, and you'll find your harvests are more abundant. Plant marigolds in close proximity to help keep pests at bay.

- **Tomatoes**—Tomatoes are among the easiest plants to grow, whether on the porch or patio or in the garden, and when harvested after being allowed to ripen on the vine, they taste absolutely fantastic. Try growing heirloom varieties for even better flavor, and if space is an issue, consider growing a crop of cherry tomatoes in a hanging planter. Keep picking them as they ripen, and your plants will continue producing delicious tomatoes all summer long.

- **Carrots**—Carrots are easy to grow in pots filled with sandy soil as well as directly in the ground. Sow a small amount of carrot seeds each week during the spring for a steady supply of fresh carrots, and if you live in a fairly warm area, you may also be able to grow fresh carrots during the winter months.

- **Cucumbers**—Cucumbers are very easy to grow, and their vines are quite attractive, making them a favorite for adding to container gardens. If you're low on garden space and are trying to decide what to grow, install a trellis and allow your cucumbers to climb it. Choose a slicing variety rather than a pickling variety when selecting seeds—these tend to have lighter flavors and smoother skins for easy handling.

- **Zucchini and Summer Squash**—So easy to grow that gardeners often find themselves passing extras out to friends and neighbors, zucchini and summer squash varieties such as crookneck and patty pan are excellent for smoothies. They're also fantastic in baked goods and when added to soups and other recipes. Grow just a few plants, allowing them to climb on trellises to save space and make harvesting easier.

- **Grapes and Fruit Trees**—Beautiful additions to landscaping and easy to maintain once established, grapevines and fruit trees can serve as a major source of delicious, almost cost-free fresh food. Be sure to find out which varieties grow well in the area where you live, and take measures to protect against birds, deer, and other animals that enjoy fruit. You can purchase fruit trees and grape vines in catalogues as well as at local nurseries. If you're not sure how to care for a tree, consider taking a class from your local garden club; you can also seek assistance from a friend, family member, or neighbor with experience.

There are many other fruits and vegetables that make excellent additions to the garden; if you are inexperienced, start small to avoid becoming overwhelmed and gain experience with organic gardening techniques. There are many fantastic books available on the topic, and there is an abundance of information available online, including websites where experienced gardeners freely share their knowledge with others. Whether you have room for a backyard garden or simply grow a few plants in containers on your porch or patio, you'll find that "growing your own" is a wonderfully rewarding experience and a great way to enjoy an abundance of healthy food.

If you don't wish to grow a garden or cannot do so, do the next best thing if possible—buy fresh produce from a local source. Small farmers typically use as little pesticide and herbicide as they can, partly because it is costly and partly because they have a vested interest in serving their communities by providing healthy food to consumers. Visit your local farmers' market, join a produce co-op that offers weekly deliveries, or look for locally grown options at the supermarket. In many places, it's also possible to visit the farms themselves, pick your own produce, and interact with the people who are responsible for growing the food that you eat.

References

Dobbins, Lee Anne. *Healthy Smoothie Recipes: Healthy Herbal Smoothies That Are Nutritious, Delicious, and Easy to Make.* Lee Anne Dobbins, 2012. Kindle.

Morris, Julie. *Superfood Kitchen: Cooking With Nature's Most Amazing Foods.* New York, NY: Sterling Epicure, 2012. Print.

Pratt, Steven G., M.D., and Kathy Matthews. *Super Foods Rx: Fourteen Foods that Will Change Your Life.* New York, NY: Harper-Collins E-books, 2012. Kindle.

Raiz, Gabrielle. *Green Smoothie Magic: More Than 132 Delicious, Adaptable Green Smoothie Recipes Using Easy to Find Ingredients.* Gabrielle Raiz, 2012. Kindle.

Rockridge University Press. *The Smoothie Recipe Book: 150 Smoothie Recipes Including Smoothies for Weight Loss and Smoothies for Good Health.* Berkeley, CA: Rockridge Press, 2013. Kindle.

Romana, Maria Elizabeth, and Beth Spicer. *Food, Glorious Food: The Kindle Carb & Calorie Counter, A Complete Guide to Food Counts.* Durham, NC: TrianglePubs.com, 2011. Kindle.

Watson, Christine. *500 Smoothies and Juices: The Only Smoothies and Juices Compendium You'll Ever Need.* Portland, ME: Sellers Publishing, Inc., 2011. Kindle.

Index

E

Eggnog, Holiday, 142
Eggplant, 157
Energy boosters, 109–123
  Berry-Almond Body
    Builder, 111
  Berry-Vanilla Vitality, 116
  Extra-Berry Energy, 117
  Green Gumption, 118
  Mango-Peach Supreme,
    120–121
  Peachy Banana Protein
    Power, 114–115
  Purple Protein
    Pick-Me-Up, 113
  Spirulina Power
    Punch, 119
  Tropical Muscle
    Machine, 112
  Veggie Verve, 122–123
Essential fatty acids, 12–13
Exercise, 50
Extra-Berry Energy, 117

F

Fermented foods, 34
Fiber, 6
Figs
  Honey-Banana Health
    Fix, 59
Filling Avocado Freeze, 72
Flavonoids, 31
Flaxseed, 12, 14, 34, 66
  Banana-Avocado
    Tummy Tamer, 90
  Breakfast of
    Champions, 68
  Cherry Champion, 137
  Hearty Banana-Flax
    Power Shake, 66
Fresh produce, versus
  frozen produce, 25

Fruits. *See also* specific
  consuming rainbow
    of, 31
  freezing fresh, 28
  picking, 29–32
  ripening naturally, 27
Fruit trees, 160
Fruity Tofu Scramble, 67

G

Garlic
  Veggie Power, 105
Ginger, 129
  Ginger Detox Delight, 129
Goji berries, 36, 58
  Pomegranate
    Protection, 71
  Tropical Muscle
    Machine, 112
Gorgeous Green Machine,
  104
Grapefruit, 158
  Carrot Cleanse, 128
  Detox Dream, 136
Grape juice
  Purple Cow, 149
Grapes, 23, 26, 155, 160
  Acai Anti-Aging
    Shake, 82
  Green Grape
    Greatness, 97
  Green Gumption, 118
  Kiwi-Banana Belly
    Blaster, 92
  Pomegranate
    Protection, 71
  Purple Cow, 149
  Purple Grape–Papaya
    Protection, 76
Greek Protein Punch, 88
Greek yogurt, 33
  Banana-Avocado
    Tummy Tamer, 90

Blueberry-Avocado
  Body Bliss, 75
Filling Avocado
  Freeze, 72
Greek Protein Punch, 88
Mindful Melon, 89
Ravishing Raspberry
  Ripple, 77–78
Green Banana Detox, 134
Green bell peppers
  Veggie Power, 105
  Veggie Verve, 122–123
Green Berry Detox Blast, 127
Green Coconut Colada, 106
Green Grape Greatness, 97
Green Gumption, 118
Green Love Machine, 99–100
Greens, 158–159
  storage of, 96
Green smoothies, 95–108
  Cucumber-Celery
    Power Cleanse,
    101–102
  Gorgeous Green
    Machine, 104
  Green Coconut
    Colada, 106
  Green Grape
    Greatness, 97
  Green Love Machine,
    99–100
  Mango Spinach
    Splash, 108
  Melon Mind Meld, 103
  Protective Peaches and
    Greens, 98
  Spiced Apple, 107
  Veggie Power, 105
Green tea, 132
  Detox Dream, 136
  Gorgeous Green
    Machine, 104
  Green Banana Detox, 134
  Green Grape
    Greatness, 97

CPSIA information can be obtained
at www.ICGtesting.com
Printed in the USA
LVOW08s0300110117
520534LV00001B/22/P